SUDDENLY A CAREGIVER
A guide to help you
through the unexpected responsibility
of caregiving

By
Darryl Pendergrass

*****

Published by Darryl Pendergrass

IBSN
978-0-9891396-0-1 (eBook)
978-0-9891396-1-8 (Paperback)

Dedication

This book is dedicated Jo Lynne Pendergrass, a life that touched the lives of many people through her display of courage in the face of adversity as she faced her battle with glioblastoma multiforme, a stage 4 brain cancer.

Acknowledgements

I want to thank my family and friends, those that came along side of Lynne and me to provide encouragement as we walked through this path of our life. I want to thank those that encouraged me to write about the experience and those that provided suggestions about the content of this book. I am deeply grateful to you. I am especially mindful of my children, Joshua and Jessica, who faced trials beyond what many must face and for their continued pain of losing their mother.

I want to thank Mari-Jo for providing ideas, support, encouragement, and the time for the writing of this book.

I also want to thank the many people who openly shared their learning about self-publishing.

Trademarks

The following products are referenced in this book. The use of these names does not imply that the trademark owners did sponsor , affiliate, or endorse this book.

AVASTIN® is a registered trademark of Genentech, Inc.
GLIADEL® Wafer is a registered trademark of Eisai Inc.
TEMODAR® is a registered trademark of Merck Sharp & Dohme Corp.

Contents

Preface

This book captures the story of a couple facing the grim reality of cancer. Through the journey, we received a crash course about what was truly important in our lives and to face each day one by one. I want to share this experience with others in the hope that at least one person is encouraged and strengthened when facing a similar situation. I want you to understand that you are not alone. While no two situations follow an exact path, I hope you draw courage, strength, and encouragement where the paths do cross.

Our lives affect the lives of other people in many ways. I hope that, more often in positive than negative ways but we learn from each other either way. We draw strength from one another and we can learn from the mistakes of others. Lynne and I were fortunate to have a strong family on both sides of our marriage and a large number of friends, so our learning experiences proved abundant. On the other side, our experience provided a learning environment for those that we interacted with during this time.

Chapter 1
Early Life

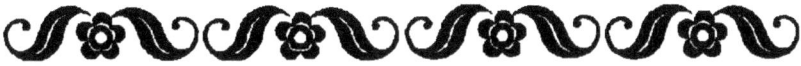

Jo Lynne was born on the evening of Wednesday, June 1, 1960 to Charles and Jean Brence in Eugene, Oregon. She lived there until she was 13 years old when job prospects caused the family to move to Scottsdale, Arizona in 1973. Lynne had two older siblings her sister, Leslie and her brother, Chuck.

I was born in 1961 in Fresno, California and moved to Scottsdale, Arizona in 1975. My dad changed career paths, moving from manufacturing and quality to that of a Church of Christ preacher, which led us to Arizona. The first Sunday of this new experience Lynne and I met for the first time. Throughout our marriage, she often laughed about that awkward, 14-year-old boy reaching out his hand to greet her and boldly saying, "Hi, I am Darryl Pendergrass."

We spent most of our teen years together spending time with other teenagers at church events. Eventually, our interest in one another surfaced. While each of us dated other people, I think we both believed deep down that we were right for each other. We wished to spend the rest of our lives together. Lynne and I married on September 7, 1979 in a ceremony, officiated by my dad, at the Scottsdale Church of Christ.

A few months later, Lynne and I decided to move to California. I based this decision on the invalid assumption that California was home despite the move to Scottsdale. One lesson I learned was that home is more about family than physical location. I worked as a journeyman grocery clerk, a job that paid well for the time but did not fulfill the needs of my personality.

I shared with Lynne that I wanted to enter the U.S. Army to learn a technical trade. I met with a recruiter and enlisted with a six-month deferment. Shortly before my induction, we moved back to Scottsdale where Lynne would live while I attended basic training at Fort Dix, New Jersey. After basic training, we moved to Aurora, Colorado so I could attend my advance training at Lowry Air Force Base.

We lived in Aurora, Colorado for about 14 months and during that time our first child, Joshua, was born. Lynne valued being a mother and caring for our baby boy. One goal of ours was to position ourselves so that she could be a stay-at-home mom.

Eventually, I received orders to Germany. I shipped out to Frankfurt for in-processing. While at Frankfurt, I learned that I would be assigned to the Fliegerhorst Kaserne just outside of Hanau and about 30 kilometers from Frankfurt. As a low ranking enlisted person, the pay was low so locating suitable off-base housing was a struggle; however, I eventually located a second story flat in town. I requested the delivery of our household goods and sent for Lynne and Joshua. The process of looking for an apartment, saving money, and the arrival of the family took about 11 months.

We settled into our new home and enjoyed our stay in Germany. We lived in Germany for three years and managed to travel to a few other countries while living there. During the final year of our stay, our daughter Jessica was born. We both cherished the ability to live among the German people and experience the culture. Long after returning home, we often talked and reminisced about our time and experience together there.

In 1985, my tour with the U.S. Army ended. We then returned to Scottsdale, Arizona so I could find new work. While in the Army, I worked as a calibration specialist – an electronics specialty. Within two weeks of returning to Scottsdale, I received an offer to work at Motorola. I quickly accepted, fulfilling a career desire that had surfaced as a young boy.

Lynne and I made Arizona our home for the remainder of our time together. We attended the Scottsdale Church of Christ and subsequently the Sun Valley Church of Christ. I served as a deacon at both congregations with Lynne working closely at my side. Lynne enjoyed entertaining and serving people so our home was often filled with friends from church. We worked diligently in the service of others. When Lynne was not entertaining, she dedicated her time to her passion of arts and crafts.

Lynne was a very industrious person. Although she never worked outside the home full-time after we married, she developed talents in various types of arts and crafts. This led to her ability to earn spending money, while working from home. She delved into many areas including tole painting and scrapbooking. Tole painting is a decorative painting folk art. Her tole painting talents led to many requests by others that she teach them techniques of the art. For several years, our living room was an art studio and training facility to many people while they learned these techniques from Lynne.

During that time, I was the envy of my work friends because for about three years, when a birthday or Christmas rolled around, buying gifts for Lynne was a breeze. She wanted power tools! (Insert Tim the Tool Man manly grunt here). I indulged her with scroll saws, band saws, drills, sanders, and other assorted tools that helped her with her crafts. When I shared the story of each gift with my friends, I received an eye roll accompanied by the statement, "You are one lucky man."

When her attention turned to scrapbooking, Lynne plunged headlong. Her nature dictated that she did nothing half-way. People often consulted her about techniques, and once again, she hosted scrapbooking parties in our home, where many friends would gather to have fun while they created their memory pages together. More than once, people joked about Lynne's scrapbooking supply room, which resembled a small store. The organization of that supply room was the opposite extreme of my home office. Her attention to detail was the butt of jokes from friends and family for years. That attention to detail spilled over into nearly everything that Lynne set her mind towards mastering or accomplishing.

Lynne loved spending time with her close friends and sharing her talents with others. She also enjoyed learning from and exchanging arts and craft ideas with others. She loved being a mother and the responsibility of caring for and raising our children. Much of her time was dedicated to ensuring their well-being, training, and entertainment.

Bad is never good until worse happens.

~Danish Proverb

Chapter 2
The Diagnosis

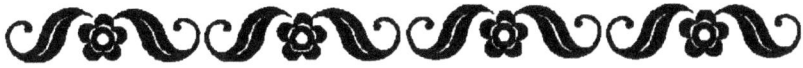

Lynne became symptomatic about a week before her diagnosis. She decided to go shopping at a local mall. Upon arrival, she opened the door of the Yukon Denali and spun herself around in the seat to exit. She slid from the seat and as her feet hit the ground, she noticed that her right leg buckled back or hyperextended. While that bothered her, she was able to continue with her shopping. Later that evening, during dinner, Lynne shared with me what had happened to her. At the time, neither of us gave much thought to what had happened, but as the week progressed additional strange symptoms occurred.

A day or two later she noticed some small tremors in her right arm and right leg. She shared each event with me as she became more concerned with each new seemingly small symptom. One evening I witnessed a seizure shortly after going to bed. The seizure was of sufficient strength to concern us both. Therefore, the next day we called her neurologist to discuss these symptoms. Due to a previous surgery to repair a degenerative disc in her neck, the neurologist requested that we come into his office later that afternoon. Since pressure on the spinal cord could produce the symptoms that we noticed, the doctor ordered an MRI (Magnetic Resonance Imaging) scan of her neck. The MRI images and associated report confirmed that a disk was compressing the spinal cord slightly.

The neurologist conferred with a neurosurgeon associate. The neurosurgeon recommended that we visit his office on the following Monday. He also suggested that we call his message service if symptoms worsened during the weekend. On Sunday morning, Lynne awoke and began her morning routine to get ready for church services. She reached for her toothbrush and added toothpaste. As she began to move the toothbrush to her mouth, she became frightened because she was unable to coordinate a movement that most of us take for granted every day. The hand holding the toothbrush seems to stop about a foot from her mouth each time she attempted that simple movement. We decided to call the neurosurgeon for his advice. He asked that we meet him at the hospital emergency room.

Soon after arriving at the hospital emergency room, the staff performed the intake procedures and moved Lynne to a room. Shortly afterwards, the neurosurgeon arrived to meet with Lynne. The neurosurgeon reviewed the MRI scan and conducted some neurological tests. Due to the compression on her spinal cord, the doctor recommended neck surgery to repair the disk. However, he stated that the neurological tests indicated that something else was also amiss because the spinal cord compression did not explain the neurological test results. Lynne agreed to the neck surgery with the understanding that additional tests would be conducted to determine the additional causes of the symptoms she was experiencing.

Lynne was soon undergoing the necessary surgical preparations then moved to the operating room. The neck surgery lasted about two hours followed by an hour or two of post-operative observation and recovery. When she was stable, I left the hospital and returned home to rest. During the night, Lynne received another MRI scan but this time including a scan of her head.

Early the next morning I awoke and prepared to return to the hospital. Shortly before leaving, I received a phone call from Lynne. By her tone and tears, I quickly realized that something was very wrong. Through tears, Lynne said the doctor had stopped by her room to inform her that the MRI scan indicated that she had a golf ball sized tumor located in the left parietal lobe of her brain. I quickly finished getting ready and began the 30-mile trip to the hospital. My mind raced with terrible thoughts and my heart was filled with compassion for Lynne who received that terrible news alone without me present with her.

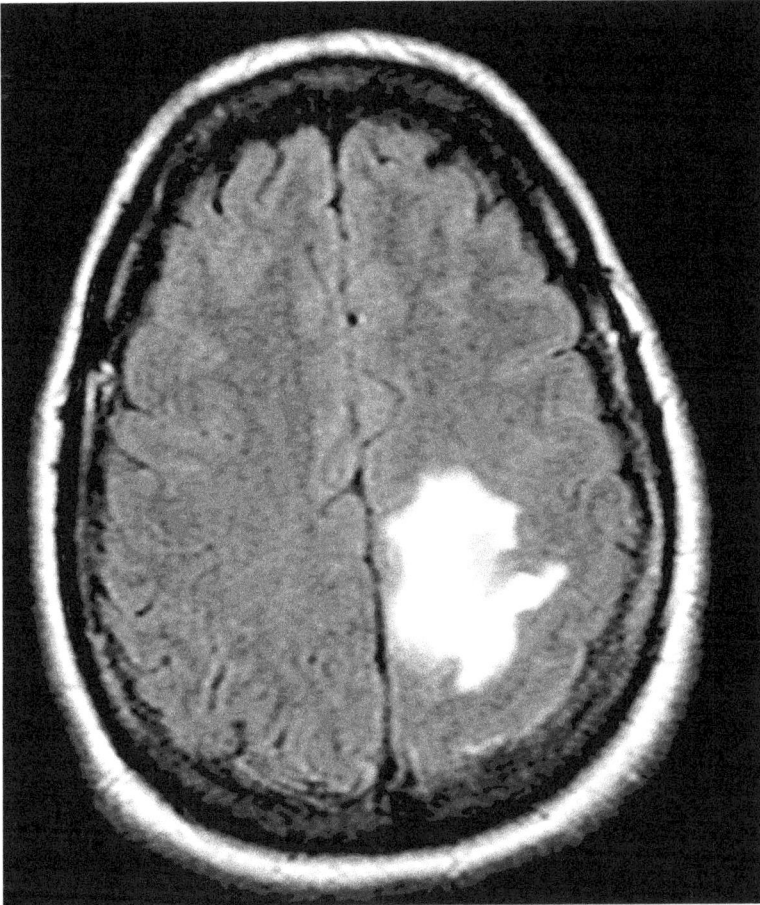

The first MRI showing the tumor located in the left parietal lobe. (Note: MRI images are reversed, so you must mentally flip the image 180°)

I arrived at the hospital. I quickly made my way to her room, where I found her still crying. I experienced the fright she must have felt at receiving this news then pondering the consequences all alone for this last hour. After what felt like an eternity, the doctor entered the room and shared two basic approaches. The first was to perform a biopsy and the second was to resect or remove the tumor. Since both approaches required invasive surgery, Lynne agreed to the resection to remove the tumor. Prior to the surgery, the surgeon again stopped by the room and we were able to discuss the situation in additional detail. Based on his experience, he believed the tumor was a type referred to as glioblastoma multiforme but admitted that only the biopsy would confirm that suspicion. He shared the risks associated with invasive brain surgery, which only added to emotions and fear that Lynne and I were harboring.

Soon, the hospital staff wheeled Lynne to the operating room. By the time the surgery began, a large group of about 30 family and friends arrived to support us while we awaited the outcome of the procedure. Nearly four hours later, the surgeon walked to the waiting room to share the news with us. He said that the procedure went as expected without complication but that determining the real effects of the surgery would require more waiting. Shortly after that, one of the nurses emerged from the recovery area to escort me to Lynne's side.

Lynne became responsive as the effects of the anesthesia wore off. One risk of the surgery included memory loss. The realization that Lynne might not recognize her family following the surgery was more terrifying to her than the surgery itself. She must have thought about that subconsciously during the surgery because as soon as the effects of the anesthesia wore off to a level that allowed her to speak, she immediately began rattling off the names of her family, "Darryl, Joshua, Jessica, and daddy."

While we were grateful that her memory remained intact, we soon realized that she was immobile on the right side of her body unable to move her right arm, leg, and toes. The hospital staff prepared us to expect a long recovery through the rehabilitation process. During Lynne's stay in the surgical recovery room, her fighting spirit soon became evident when the nurse asked her to move her right toes. Unable to, she slyly slid the left foot covered by the blankets close enough to the right foot to move the toes. The nurse laughed and accused Lynne of "cheating," causing Lynne and I to chuckle as well.

Three days after her first brain surgery the results from the pathology test arrived. The neurosurgeon confirmed his suspicion that the tumor was indeed a stage 4 brain tumor referred to as glioblastoma multiforme. With those results in hand, my analytical nature kicked into high gear. I researched for several hours that afternoon and evening to learn all that I could about this disease. The statistics were dire. One report stated that left untreated, most patients would die within six months. With treatment, the prognosis was not much better with most patients dying within 18 months. My job responsibilities included training as a Six Sigma black belt, which included analyzing data and applying statistical techniques for decision-making. I realized that statistics are useful for analyzing groups but held onto the hope that these numbers would not apply to Lynne – an individual case, a person. Despite my state of shock and dismay, I shared the information with the family so all would recognize the severity of the challenges that lie ahead, but I also consoled them and myself that each case depends on individual circumstances. Lynne was young and otherwise healthy. The statistics indicated that the largest group of people with this disease was Caucasian men over 70 years of age.

For the first few days of Lynne's stay in the urgent care, she was comfortable staying alone so family members returned home during the evenings to rest. However, one night, in between nurse checks, the nurse call button fell between the mattress and the hospital bed frame on her right side. Since her right side was immobile, the inability to call the nurse frightened her to a state of panic. From that night on, she requested that a family member stay with her. Some of us shared that duty each night, for the remainder of her hospital stay.

Lynne recovered quickly enough from the surgery to begin the transition from the hospital to a resident therapy facility. The doctors, nurses, and social workers worked with us to prepare us for the days that lie ahead. Following the surgery and inpatient rehabilitation, Lynne would require about 30 days of radiation treatments followed by 30 days of chemotherapy treatments.

The most important thing in illness is never to lose heart.
~Nikolai Lenin

Chapter 3
The Treatments

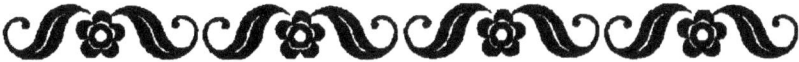

Just a few days after the brain surgery to remove the golf ball-sized tumor from Lynne's left parietal lobe, the hospital staff organized and transported Lynne to the inpatient rehabilitation facility. After the initial assessments, the staff suggested that the rehabilitation could take up to three months.

Moving to the facility was a shock for Lynne and me. At 46, Lynne was the youngest patient. People 20 to 30 years her senior filled the facility suffering mostly from strokes. I noticed this affected Lynne most drastically when all patients gathered in the common dining room for breakfast, lunch, and dinner. I could sense the pain in her eyes as she realized the gravity of her situation at such a young age.

Therapists scheduled sessions for short blocks of time each day for physical, occupational, and speech therapy. Each session took a toll on Lynne. Despite her frustration about not being able to do simple tasks that most of us take for granted (even she herself just a few days earlier), Lynne focused and worked diligently at every challenge presented to her by the therapists.

I remember the first session that began on her second day at the facility like an indelible image burned into my memory. The staff moved Lynne from her bed to a wheelchair and wheeled her to the corridor just outside her room. We had already learned that the goal of rehabilitation was not necessarily to make someone complete again but simply to make them functional and to relearn basic tasks that created some semblance of independence. I stood behind her, as she sat in the chair with the therapist providing her instructions. He wanted her to wheel herself down the corridor. She listened intently then moved her left arm to the wheel and the left foot to the floor. The therapist moved her immobile right arm to the wheel and her immobile right leg to the floor. With the focus of an excellent athlete, Lynne gave her all to move the wheelchair though the corridor. I returned to her room, with my eyes filled with tears, where I met her father who also had eyes filled with tears. The tears were two fold, one because of the example of courage we both just witnessed but also because of the realization of what had happened in our lives.

After the session, the therapists helped Lynne back to the room and made her comfortable in her bed. She informed me beyond any doubt that she would be out of the facility in two weeks not three months as suggested by the therapy staff. That determination drove Lynne to work each day on every task assigned, although sometimes with tears from pure frustration and exhaustion.

The therapists and nurses caring for Lynne shared that she inspired them because of her determination and charm. One of the night nurses enjoyed Lynne's optimistic personality despite the tragic events that Lynne now faced. One morning, the nurse brought in a beautiful glass display with the words of the serenity prayer engraved. That gift provided inspiration to Lynne and me for many months to come and still sits in my room as a reminder that we do not control everything that happens in our lives.

God, grant me the serenity to accept the things I
cannot change,
the courage to change the things I can,
and the wisdom to know the difference.

The family also received training about techniques for helping Lynne and ensuring her safety once Lynne returned home. Lynne's persistence paid off because in just eight days, Lynne received news that the therapists believed Lynne was ready to return home.

The 22-mile drive home seemed like a lifetime for Lynne, but she was very thankful to step through the garage door into the kitchen of our home. Lynne was able to do much on her own but required assistance at every step just to ensure her safety. Lynne underwent physical therapy at home, three times per week, to continue to build her strength and independence.

The day after she arrived home, she was able to curl the toes on her right foot for the first time since the brain surgery. While a simple thing for most of us, this was monumental event for Lynne.

The number of cards and gifts that Lynne received over the first two weeks of this ordeal humbled us both. The cards and gifts continued to arrive regularly over the next couple of months. Each expression gave Lynne and me encouragement to face each day. Two or three wise people also sent cards of encouragement to me directly. I encourage you to remember not only the patient but also those that care for them.

Two or three wise people also sent cards of encouragement to me directly. I encourage you to remember not only the patient but also those that care for them.

While Lynne was in the rehabilitation facility, the staff often shared information about the disease for our learning. The speech therapist shared information about a particularly insightful event about brain cancer scheduled for the first Saturday following Lynne's return to home. While the family cared for Lynne, I attended the event at Barrow's Neurological Institute in downtown Phoenix, Arizona. A good portion of the seminar focused on the specific type of cancer that Lynne was battling. The seminar included the topics 1) diagnosis (MRI and pathology), 2) neurosurgery, 3) chemotherapy, 4) radiation, 5) research updates, 6) quality of life issues, including caregiver information, and 7) a mock tumor board meeting. There was more information provided than I could possibly absorb in one day. I was thankful to have the reference material so that we could learn about the various issues we were to face. The statistics that I discovered relating to survival from this cancer were bleak. I was encouraged to meet a middle-aged man at the seminar who was a 13-year survivor of a glioblastoma tumor located and treated in his temporal lobe. I used that information to reinforce with the family that hope does exist despite the dreary statistics.

And hope does not disappoint us, because God has poured out his love into our hearts by the Holy Spirit, whom he has given us.
Roman 5:5

Lynne returned to the hospital just twelve days following her return home due to pain in her chest. Tests indicated that she had a blood clot in her right lung. They also discovered that the right leg was full of clots and the left ankle had a clot. The five days spent in the hospital dampened Lynne's spirits some but her jovial spirit returned, as did her beautiful smile. Despite this difficulty in her life, those traits inspired those around her.

Since the brain surgery, Lynne received many medications to control swelling of the brain, which often caused seizures induced by the tumor and surgery. Monitoring was crucial to ensure the medication levels stayed within range. Levels that were too low were not therapeutic and levels that were too high could be fatal. For the most part, the levels stayed within range but occasionally would fall below or above range causing fear and trips to the emergency room. Medicine interactions often complicated the situation.

One month following the brain surgery, Lynne had a follow up MRI scan. The results were much less than we had hoped for, since the tumor area still showed about a 13 millimeter sized area of active tumor. Glioblastoma Multiforme is known for its fast growth and recurrence properties, which is something I learned during my research, but now was learning from reality. We learned at a subsequent neurosurgeon appointment that the image showed residual tumor and not new growth. This was point of learning for me and awareness of why the term physician practice is used. I learned that doctors attending to patients rotate shifts and often have only cursory awareness of each patient's condition and history. Therefore, it became important to seek as much information as possible and seek second or third opinions if needed.

During that hospital stay, the staff began the process of preparing for the radiation treatments. On the first day, Lynne was fitted with a mesh mask that would secure her head while in the treatment. She was extremely claustrophobic and terror filled her when they affixed the mask for the practice run. The staff was very accommodating and trimmed as much from the mask as possible to reduce her fears. I also talked with her and encouraged her to face this fear to allow the radiation to proceed and help minimize the possibility of the tumor recurring.

Lynne was a true animal lover. She and I were both raised on farms, so each of us was familiar with animals. She really enjoyed having cats and dogs in the house. During the often-long stays in the hospital, she received several visits from pet therapy people. Even if she was unable to speak due to swelling in the brain, she still smiled broadly each time she received a visit by a pet. I send a big thank you to all of you who volunteer your time performing this role, thank you.

I send a big thank you to those who volunteer their time as pet therapists

Upon her return home, she often felt nauseated and dizzy. We discovered that this is common after being somewhat sedentary in the hospital. To assist her recovery, the family shared responsibility to ensure that every two hours she was up and walking about. I purchased some new patio furniture so we could spend some time outside relaxing and talking. She enjoyed the sound of birds and the water fountain more than ever before. I could tell that a new appreciation of life was building within Lynne. In our ever increasingly fast-paced world, we often become numb to the little things in life that are most familiar to us. We also tend to forget the simple things that can bring joy into our lives. When we believe we will live forever, we often miss those little things because we pursue even less meaningful things in life or as Stephen Covey suggests, we often pursue the urgent rather than important things in our life.

Finally, brothers, whatever is true, whatever is noble, whatever is right, whatever is pure, whatever is lovely, whatever is admirable—if anything is excellent or praiseworthy—think about such things.

Philippians 4:8

The radiation treatments began. Following a rough day during the practice run, I was wary that she would be able to complete the first treatment. Lynne did pull together the courage to face her claustrophobia. As I watched the treatment through a video monitor, I was proud of Lynne's determination beyond my ability to express in words. At this point in our lives, we had been married for 28 years, but, until that moment, I had underestimated everything that made Lynne truly special.

For six weeks, the family rotated duties for transporting Lynne to the hospital for radiation treatments, a 60-mile round trip, which required most of the morning to complete. Toward the end of the radiation treatments, we noticed that Lynne tired more easily partly due to the radiation treatments and partly due to the schedule demands of the last month.

After six weeks, the radiation treatments were finished and the chemotherapy began. The chemotherapy chosen was Temodar®, a newer drug that showed promising results for this type of brain cancer. Nausea is one of the frequently published side effects of many chemotherapy medications. We learned all about that in the wee hours of the morning following her first dose of the drug. Since these treatments were planned to last a year, we were glad to discover that the nausea medication prescribed – just in case – was effective in reducing the nausea to a manageable level in about 30 minutes, but what a 30 minutes - dry heaves that increased the pressure on her already sensitive brain causing a severe headache.

The first two months following Lynne's brain surgery included several trips back to the hospital for one reason or another. Finally, her progress began to be visible to her. She began walking unassisted. One afternoon following her release from the hospital to regulate her Phenytoin levels, she walked to the bedroom. Several minutes later, I decided to check on her and found her sitting on the edge of the bathtub filing her fingernails. She just looked up at me and smiled. I realized that she was enjoying her alone time following two months of someone always being at her side, watching her every move. This was an important lesson for me as a caregiver. Just two short months ago, Lynne was fully independent and losing that independence is a difficult inner struggle. So when safe to do so, I tried to provide Lynne with treasured alone time to increase her sense of independence. Lynne also began returning to the kitchen to help with meal preparation. Cooking was a passion for Lynne, especially baking. On the third night that she assisted with the preparation of the evening meal, she confided in me that she believed she was on her way to recovery. I welcomed that news after the inner turmoil of the last two months.

I realized that she was enjoying her alone time following two months of someone always being at her side, watching her every move. This was an important lesson for me as a caregiver.

Three months following Lynne's initial brain surgery, a friend from Connecticut arrived to spend a long weekend with Lynne. We first met Joyce over a decade earlier when she and her husband lived in Arizona. We attended church together and became close friends. Work eventually moved the family to Connecticut and for many years, we had little to no contact. We reconnected during Lynne's illness. That friendship led to several additional visits to spend time with Lynne. Those visits were typically filled with laughter, sharing memories, and helping Lynne. A huge benefit that I observed was that Lynne was able to be *normal* for a change, not focused on her terminal illness.

The first nine months were filled with doctor visits nearly every week, several return trips to the hospital to address complications, and MRI scans to track the condition of the tumor following the brain surgery, radiation, and chemotherapy. Nevertheless, Lynne's condition did stabilize enough to allow Lynne to return to some semblance of a normal life.

Fifteen months after her diagnosis, an MRI scan indicated a concern including the possibility of recurrent cancer. We met with the neurosurgeon for guidance. He described the recurrence as minimal but suggested that we confer with the Barrow Neurological Institute (BNI) about a Gamma Knife procedure. The Barrow Neurological Institute is a world-renowned treatment center. We were grateful to have such a facility located within driving distance of our home. The BNI houses the only Gamma Knife facility in the state – at least at that time.

Within a month of her last MRI scan, Lynne began to experience seizures again. The doctors adjusted medication levels to control the seizures but the return of seizures after many months concerned Lynne and me. My research found that this cancer tends to recur between 9 and 15 months. At this point Lynne was at the 16-month mark since the initial detection of the tumor.

The hospital admitted Lynne to the Barrow Neurological Institute for the Gamma Knife procedure. The Gamma Knife provides a means to treat the condition non-invasively through focused radiation. The Gamma Knife uses 192 individually controllable beams of radiation. Each beam alone contains minimal radiation but when all beams focus on one area, that radiation increases dramatically. One benefit is that the procedure often requires only a single day's stay in the hospital. The recurrent tumor was not clearly defined enough to allow the neuro-oncologist to determine the extent and precise location of the treatment. The neuro-oncologist radiated as much of the recurrent tumor as possible without compromising her quality of life.

Following the Gamma Knife procedure, the oncologist recommended resuming chemotherapy using Temodar®. After the first chemotherapy treatment following her initial brain surgery, the oncologist abandoned subsequent treatments because Lynne's platelet levels had dropped to near fatal levels. The low platelet levels required that Lynne undergo a blood transfusion to correct the issue. The chemotherapy maintenance program consisted of the oral medication each day for a week followed by three weeks of no medication to allow the body to recover. Despite the previous experience with chemotherapy, Lynne and I agreed to resume the maintenance program because Glioblastoma Multiforme demonstrates aggressive growth and recurrence properties. The first night resulted in several hours of dry heaving before the nausea settled enough for Lynne to rest. The next day we spoke with the oncologist who agreed to provide a stronger medication to counteract the nausea effects caused by the chemotherapy.

Following the resumption of the chemotherapy maintenance program, Lynne's blood white count level plunged. The doctor prescribed her a self-administered injection designed to boost the white count level. The low white count level also required that Lynne avoid crowds, frequent hand washing, and cooking foods thoroughly to prevent infections. Even after one month, blood tests indicated levels outside of the normal range that required the use of additional medications to strengthen Lynne's immune system. The treatments required another week of the self-administered shots to boost her system.

Lynne's doctor ordered another MRI scan to track the progress of the tumor. Two months after the Gamma Knife procedure, the MRI scan results showed stability compared to the two previous results. The next MRI scan taken four months after the Gamma Knife procedure showed enhancement of the tumor once again and a slight change in shape but did not indicate any sign of aggressive growth.

Lynne continued to receive MRI scans nearly every two months for the remainder of her life. As the time approached for a scan so did the anxiety about the results. Depending on the treatment regimen, the tumor might have decreased, a welcomed result, or growth that caused increased stress about the next set of treatments that might ensue.

The first eight months of 2009 were good for Lynne. The MRI scans, every two months, showed the tumor was stable and treatments were minimal. However, the August scan showed a concern leading to the BNI neurosurgeon recommending another brain surgery to explore the tumor area. Due to the previous brain surgery, radiation, and the Gamma Knife procedure, it was becoming increasingly difficult to separate scar tissue from tumor growth using the MRI scan alone. In early September, Lynne underwent the second invasive brain surgery. The surgery lasted about three and a half hours. The neurosurgeon reported that he removed as much as he felt he could safely remove without inducing additional deficits in her motor skills.

Lynne returned home just three days after her second invasive brain surgery. However, just a week later, she returned to the emergency room with a severe bout of seizures. Her right side also lost most of its mobility. The mobility returned within a couple of days, allowing her to return home. The doctors believed that swelling (edema) in the brain combined with a low level of seizure medication caused the seizures.

The physical rehabilitation resumed to build her strength. We traveled to a nearby rehabilitation center two or three times per week depending on Lynne's ability. The therapy alternated between physical therapy and occupational therapy. The physical therapy focused on building strength and coordination for walking. The occupational therapy focused on strengthening the arms and rebuilding the coordination lost due to the brain surgery.

Lynne once again resumed chemotherapy. Because Lynne did not respond well to the side effects of the Temodar® regimen previously administered, the oncologist recommended a combination of Avastin® and Irinotecan. Avastin® (Bevacizumab) originally targeted metastatic colon cancer but was later targeted for other types of cancer, such as breast cancer. The FDA approved Avastin® for use with glioblastoma multiforme in May 2009. The FDA (Federal Drug Administration) removed the approval for use with breast cancer in 2011 but allowed to continue to use the medication for other types of cancer (Pazdur, 2011). Avastin® works by inhibiting the development of vessels that supply blood to the tumor (Genentech, 2012). Irinotecan blocks the action of an enzyme affecting the DNA causing cell death. Since cancer cells grow faster than normal cells, the probability of affecting the cancer cells is higher than that of the normal cells. (American Cancer Society, 2009). These treatments required daily trips to the oncology office. The office seated about 20 people undergoing treatments for some form of cancer. Lynne enjoyed visiting with other patients when she could and I believe that most of the patients enjoyed her positive outlook. The fatigue caused by the medications building up in her system and the frequent 60-mile round trips to the treatment facility caused Lynne to sleep for the majority of each day.

The chemotherapy continued regularly for several months. Lynne also continued to receive MRI scans every other month. The doctor encouraged her on her third year of survival. Surviving glioblastoma multiforme for this length of time placed Lynne in a small group of survivors. Only 5% of people survive through the first five years (CBTRUS, 2012). The regular MRI scans showed stability for the most part until March 2010, which indicated a subtle enhancement of the tumor. Her next MRI scan in June indicated evidence of nodular enhancement and a thin rind of enhancement along the entire periphery of the tumor resection cavity. No evidence of midline shift was present indicating the cancer had not migrated to other parts of the brain. Midline shift referred to the cancer crossing from the left to right hemisphere of the brain. The medical team recommended action.

The neurosurgeon at the BNI suggested that Lynne might be a candidate for an experimental trial treatment. Lynne and I spoke privately at length about moving from approved and traditional treatments to experimental treatments. At this point, Lynne had already received most of the traditional and approved treatments. Lynne understood the risks and told me that if she could help someone else in the future by participating in an experiment that she would agree to the treatment. Within a few days, we discovered that she did not qualify for the study because this was the fourth recurrence of the tumor. Scientists tightly control the experiments to enhance the repeatability of the studies.

In July 2010, the BNI tumor board recommended another brain surgery followed by additional chemotherapy. Lynne was anxious but prepared for her third invasive brain surgery. The neurosurgeon suggested placing Gliadel® wafers into the resection area after the tumor removal. On surgery day, the neurosurgeon shared the results of an MRI scan from the previous day. The tumor had invaded the motor strip, which increased the surgical risk dramatically. The neurosurgeon offered two options: an aggressive or a non-aggressive procedure. The risk of the aggressive option was potentially severe paralysis on her right side. The benefit was longer life expectation. The reverse was true for the non-aggressive option. Lynne and I discussed the options. We preferred and agreed to pursue the aggressive option. With the aggressive option, the need for rehabilitation was a near certainty. The surgery lasted much longer than planned. The neurosurgeon assured me that this was not related to complications, but additional time was required due to the tumor's invasion of the motor strip. Lynne was able to move her right arm and leg during recovery, which provided a ray of hope that the paralysis would not be permanent.

Goodbyes are not forever.

Goodbyes are not the end.

They simply mean I'll miss you

Until we meet again!

~Author Unknown

Chapter 4
Saying Goodbye

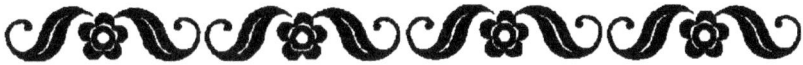

In retrospect, the third invasive brain surgery – 41 months into her battle – marked the steady decline in Lynne's quality of life. Up to that point, despite the battle, Lynne maintained a good quality of life. During her hospital recovery, she had extreme difficulty verbalizing her thoughts and struggled to assemble full sentences. I could sense the frustration she held because of the inability to communicate effectively. The need for physical, occupational, and speech therapy was extensive. I did my best to reassure her but I could sense that Lynne was showing signs of exhaustion from the three-year ordeal.

The nurses shared with me the pleasure they received when caring for Lynne. Lynne never failed to say "thank you" for even the most simple of requests. She received therapy during her hospital stay but remained frustrated and emotional due to the inability to express her thoughts. There were times when she could speak so I suspected that increasing and decreasing amounts of swelling in her brain were playing a part.

For the first time, I witnessed discouragement and her preparation to end her fight. Her emotional frustration continued with the increased deficiencies she experienced in her right arm and leg coupled with the difficulty in expressing her thoughts and concerns. Seizures resumed in her right side causing much discomfort. She managed to tell me, "You should throw me out." A statement like that from Lynne was very out of character for her.

Sensing her pain, I assured her that I did not intend to forsake my love and responsibility to her.

A visit from the neurosurgeon indicated that much of the tumor enhancement was de-bulked during the surgery but he was not hopeful for much improvement in her physical condition because of the progression of the cancer into the motor strip. One afternoon, she managed to say, "Get me outta here" so we located a wheelchair and moved her to a window view. Getting out of the confined space of the hospital room was enough to lift her spirits a bit until the exhaustion of the brief trip caused her to become sleepy and ready to return to her bed.

After one week in the hospital to recover from the surgery, the staff told Lynne that she would move to an in-patient rehabilitation facility. She was all smiles and did not want any grass growing under her feet. Once the order was given, we packed the room and she was moved into an ambulance for transport within ten minutes. The Rhodes rehabilitation center moved to a new location since Lynne's last visit but there were still some familiar faces.

Lynne faced a massive task to recover some self-sufficiency and to restore her ability to communicate effectively. I believe the size of the mountain became more clearly visible for both of us. I sensed she was overwhelmed with what she knew lay ahead. Each day she completed three hours of therapy - one hour each of speech, occupational, and physical therapy. All sessions were back-to-back then lunch, so she was exhausted and ready for a nap every afternoon. The evenings were emotional for Lynne. When she was unable to express the source of her frustrations and emotions, I tried to withhold the tendency to fill in the blanks for her. I suspected the turmoil of the previous week supplied a combination of many thoughts that swirled within her mind.

When she was unable to express the source of her frustrations and emotions, I tried to withhold the tendency to fill in the blanks for her.

I made Lynne lunch and brought it up for her one day. She liked my green chili cheese enchiladas. I also made Spanish rice. After eating hospital food for a couple of weeks, I suddenly turned into a master chef in Lynne's eyes. She enjoyed the meal and I enjoyed making it for her. She was a little disturbed that I moved the cheesecake, delivered by the hospital, away from her to eat lunch first. My brother, daughter, Lynne's sister, and nephew shared the meal with us in the family room of the rehabilitation center. She enjoyed sharing time with family and friends.

Lynne's therapy progressed nicely. The therapists added one additional session to the afternoon. Her speech did not show much improvement over the week but her progress led to the decision to release her from the in-patient center and return home for continued therapy in an outpatient facility. A couple of days before her expected release from the rehabilitation center, Lynne tried to stand up without assistance and fell, hitting her left cheek on the handle next to the bathroom toilet. A CT (Computed Tomography) scan followed and did not show any extensive problems. Lynne's cheek showed signed of swelling; I expected that she would have a noticeable reminder the next day, to ensure she ask for assistance.

I noticed that this surgery limited Lynne's ability to focus on multiple conversations or compound instructions – those containing multiple steps in one sentence. While Lynne enjoyed company, I began restricting visits as they were beginning to overwhelm her causing frustration and anxiety. Her brain had to work much harder on those tasks that the rest of do without even a second thought. I began to watch more closely those that visited her to ensure that they understood the difficulty she had conversing with multiple people at the same time.

Lynne still had her sense of humor and a beautiful, contagious smile. Humor was always a part of our lives, which we enjoyed beginning in the early days of our lives together. Humor was a daily part of our routine. We even had a "rule" to laugh at least once per day. That practice proved useful now as our habit to laugh diverted our thoughts if only for a moment.

She is clothed with strength and dignity; she can laugh at the days to come.
Proverbs 31:25

One of Lynne's favorite treats was a caramel frappe. On one trip to the rehabilitation center, I stopped to pick up her favorite treat. When I arrived, she still had a couple of hours of rehabilitation to complete before I could serve it to her. I placed it into a public refrigerator and let Lynne know that the treat was waiting for her when she was finished. She worked extra hard as she now had a major reward placed before her. When the time arrived, I retrieved the treat and handed it to her. After a couple of slurps from the straw, I asked her if it was good. She gave a quite reply; she said "fantastilicous." I do not think that is a word but I was very happy to hear five syllables uttered to perfection. I thought that was just – well – *fantastilicous.*

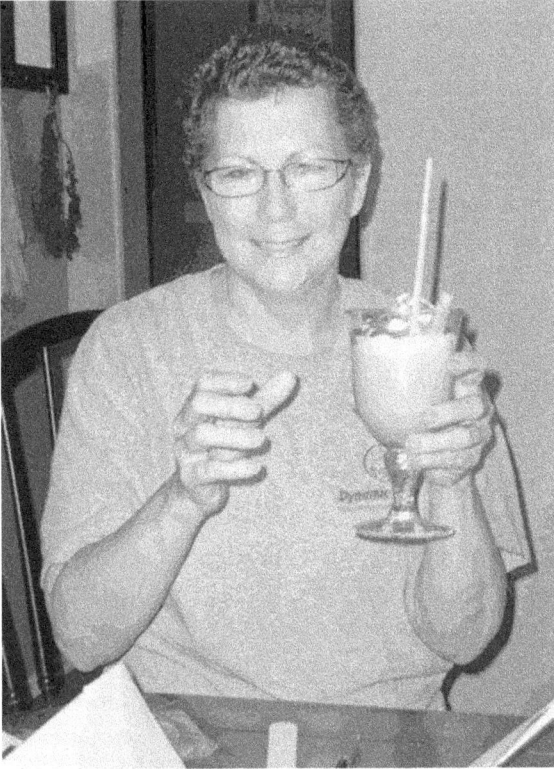

Lynne with a homemade caramel frappe

Lynne improved her strength, walking about 250 feet one day with minimal assistance and used her feet to move her wheelchair about 150 feet. At that point, Lynne participated in five to six hours of therapy per day. She enjoyed her frequent naps during the day and slept well at night. The rehabilitation doctor targeted her release at about four more days of inpatient rehabilitation then continued therapy at home. I met with a speech therapist and she was encouraged by Lynne's progress. The therapist believed Lynne understood most of what she heard and recognized objects that she saw but the connections between the brain and nerves caused her to struggle to control the mouth to speak. (I actually have observed this in many people but they do not have the same excuse that Lynne had.) I was encouraged with the progress and understood that the recovery would be somewhat lengthy. The therapist mentioned that her mother was also diagnosed with glioblastoma multiforme. Her mother passed away from a combination of issues but did do very well for a time.

As the day neared for Lynne to go home, her excitement began to grow. My daughter Jessica and I worked with the therapists to refresh our memories and share new techniques that we might need to assist Lynne at home. We practiced with Lynne entering and exiting our vehicle. Nevertheless, for the first time during this ordeal, she was unable to negotiate the steps of the Denali. We decided to use my daughter's car the next day to transport Lynne to our home. Both of the vehicles that Lynne and I owned were similar, so I needed to do some quick shopping for a replacement vehicle that I could use to move Lynne to the various appointments that followed.

During the speech therapy session that day, the speech therapist showed Lynne a variety of pictures to test her recall and remind her about the object names. One picture was of a girl in a dress that resembled something from the movie *The Sound of Music*. The expected answer was "girl" but Lynne replied "Betty Crocker." The girl's dress certainly looked like she was wearing an apron. We all chuckled, Lynne included, and I assured the therapist that given Lynne's love of cooking the answer was quite appropriate. At lunch, I noticed some of the residents were not present but also noticed several new faces. I attended nearly every lunch and dinner so noticing the changing faces was not a surprise; however, I assure you that even the unfamiliar could pick out the new residents because each of them ordered the vegetable lasagna. The experienced residents only made that mistake once.

On my way home, I stopped by a warehouse store. They had a sampling table setup with dipped apples with a variety of different coatings. I had to chuckle because about seven or eight ladies stood before the large glass counter with the "look" – you know the one that appears when chocolate is in sight. Just two aisles over another sample table presented sugar-free chocolate for sampling. The vendor standing behind the sampling table was one of the loneliest looking vendors I have ever seen at a warehouse store. I made a wise decision and opted for the apples. When Lynne called me later that evening, I shared the apple choices that were available. She requested that I bring the cherry dipped apple.

The next day I arrived at the hospital at eight o'clock in the morning. just in time to spend the last few minutes with her as she finished her breakfast. After breakfast, we met with the therapist to practice a bit by simulating the navigation of the entry way into our home and with transferring her into Jessica's car and out again. At her next rest period, I unveiled the cherry dipped apple that caused Lynne to present an ear-to-ear grin. We enjoyed our little treat to celebrate Lynne's going home party.

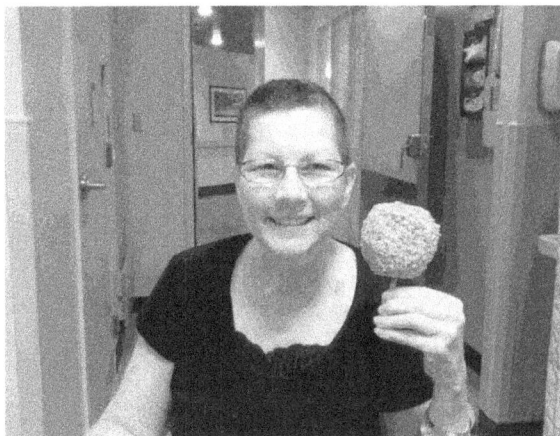

Lynne with a cherry-dipped apple

We were waiting for hospital discharge papers all morning and into the early afternoon hours. When lunchtime arrived, a nurse stuck her head into the room asking Lynne if she wanted lunch. She replied quickly, "No, Darryl is taking me out." I convinced her to eat something just to hold her over until we could make it to a restaurant of her choice. Hospitals are much like the military – hurry up and wait.

After a couple of days of searching, I located a potential vehicle that suited Lynne's needs for one that was lower to the ground, so she could get in and out safely. Given the number of doctor appointments she was scheduled for over the next few weeks, moving quickly was important.

I located a Cadillac CTS-V on a local dealer website on Friday. On Saturday, the vehicle was no longer available on the website, so I started searching for other suitable alternatives. On Sunday, much to my surprise and delight, the vehicle once again appeared on the website so I showed up at opening time for a test drive. Come to find out, a co-worker of my brother was looking at the same vehicle; luckily I beat him to the punch. He was the reason the vehicle was unavailable on the website on Saturday. On my way out the door, Lynne managed to say "Black." She loves black vehicles with chrome wheels. I assured her that I had her back on this one.

The deal was a good one. I traded in both vehicles. During the previous year, one of the trade-ins I managed to drive the vehicle only driving 1,200 miles. Nevertheless, I was thankful that the deal worked and we received the extra benefit of not paying insurance and registration on a vehicle we used so little. We had kept the vehicle just in case Lynne improved to a point where she could drive again.

So back to the CTS-V, the V included the Corvette LS6 engine and all of the performance tweaks and options one would expect from Cadillac. While I made sure that the vehicle met Lynne's needs, the horsepower and 0-60 M.P.H. time was just for me. That is what makes a good marriage right? - compromise. When I brought the vehicle home, she wanted a ride. So we moved out of the neighborhood onto a country road and I told her to put her head on the headrest. She ignored my request but as I punched the accelerator, the car convinced her to do otherwise. As I slowed down, she turned her head toward me and the eyebrows contorted into a shape that made me quite aware that she never wanted to experience that again! She could not speak but the eyebrows spoke volumes.

Our first week home was more or less uneventful. Lynne had moments where she was able to speak clearly but most of the time she struggled piecing together her thoughts into coherent speech. Lynne slept well at night, which was a relief. When I got a good night's sleep, I had much more energy throughout the day. Jessica was also contributing most of her time to ensure that Lynne had a 24-hour watch.

I coordinated doctor appointments and Lynne's continued rehabilitation therapy. The rehabilitation doctor and I agreed to pursue home therapy but the discharging physician prescribed outpatient therapy. Her primary care physician supposedly sent an order to a local home therapy company but when I called, they claimed no knowledge about receiving such an order. We met with her primary care physician to get everything corrected. Outpatient therapy was much too difficult and demanding given the other regular doctor appointments. Lynne mentioned at breakfast one morning that she was ready to get working on the rehabilitation. I also coordinated the resumption of her chemotherapy treatments. The neuro-oncologist recommended a modification in her treatment, so I greased the communication skids to ensure that her treating oncologist received the recommendation and scheduled her first appointment.

Lynne and I met with the neurosurgeon for a post-surgical checkup. He was pleased with the healing of the surgical site. Given the significant deficiencies resulting from the surgery, I asked the surgeon about the likelihood of any future surgical procedures. He confirmed my suspicion. The risk associated with each subsequent surgery increased significantly compared to the previous procedures. We will need to consider any future procedures with great care. For the future, we looked to the chemotherapy as the primary treatment.

Over the course of the next few weeks, Lynne's recovery from her surgery moved along steadily. She had nine appointments during a typical week including doctors, therapists, and home nurse visits. Following each therapy appointment, she was definitely ready for a nap. Lynne still struggled with her speech. She had moments of clear speech but often struggled to find the words to express her thoughts.

Without warning one day, the batteries for the universal entertainment system remote went bad so I had to make an emergency run to purchase the replacement AAA batteries. That was only an emergency when one was stuck on the couch most of the day. As I made my way to the garage, Lynne said, "Can I ride along?" She was already dressed and ready since she had just finished a physical therapy session. I helped her to the car for a few minutes out of the house. Once into the car, she said, "You know I have a plan." She did not have to say any more, I knew what she wanted – a caramel frappe, you know the one that is fantastilicious.

Lynne's sister was able to sit with Lynne for a few hours. Jessica went to the mall for a little breather and I got a little uninterrupted work time. Lynne looked forward to a upcoming visit from our friend from Connecticut. Lynne enjoyed those visits as she got some time to talk about things other than cancer, doctors, and treatments.

We met with the neuro-oncologist to discuss chemotherapy options. He recommended switching to bis-chloroethylnitrosourea (BCNU) due to Lynne's sensitivity to Temodar®. Lynne almost lost her life when taking Temodar® three years ago due to platelet counts that plunged to fatal levels. Temodar® is a one of the gold-standard treatments, especially following the initial diagnosis. BCNU is one of the original treatments for GBM approved by the FDA (Federal Drug Administration) in 1977. BCNU is the same agent that is in the Gliadel® wafers implanted during surgery.

Lynne resumed chemotherapy treatments about six weeks after the third invasive brain surgery. Lynne was feeling a little lethargic over the last several days so I called the doctor to order some blood work to see if anything was amiss and to ensure that her body was ready for this dose of chemotherapy. The results indicated that her blood levels were in good shape. Lynne did not have any of her regular blood lab appointments since before her last surgery. She and one of the lab managers became quite close over the last three years, since Lynne had blood drawn nearly every week or so. When we arrived, I saw some tears flow from the lab manager's eyes, as she was concerned about what had happened to Lynne because we had not been in the lab for nearly three months. Lynne touched lives no matter where her journey took her. One day a home nurse visited and at the conclusion of her visit said, "To know Lynne is to love Lynne." She reached that conclusion after only knowing Lynne for three weeks.

Joyce, our friend from Connecticut, arrived just in time for Jessica's departure to Las Vegas for a little rest and relaxation and a birthday celebration. I always enjoyed seeing what a good time Lynne and Joyce had while together. I also appreciated the help more than words could express.

During this time, my employer of 25 years announced the sale of the Motorola Networks business to Nokia Siemens Networks. The regulatory approvals were underway. I expected the acquisition to prove beneficial for both companies. I was already busy trying to understand what the acquisition meant in terms of the information systems group - no small task given the size of the corporations. Such events always provide the opportunity to learn new skills and acquire knowledge. I enjoy learning, so I looked forward to the challenge.

On September 7, 2010, Lynne and I celebrated 31 years of marriage. We had a fun day reminiscing about our life together. I treated her to a Swiss steak dinner with mashed potatoes. She requested a date to a local Mexican restaurant, but we decided to do that a few days later, as she had several therapy treatments that day. She did pause at one point in the day and wanted to propose. Of course, I said "Yes."

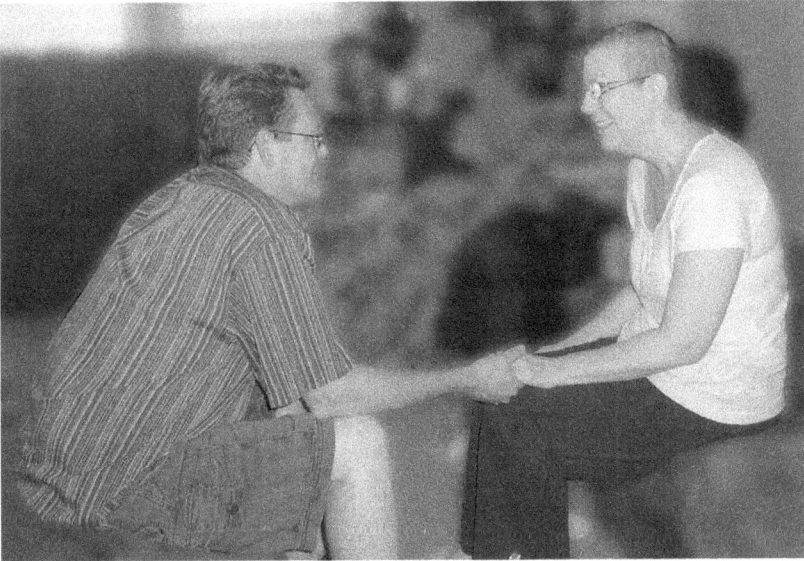

The lab results of Lynne's blood test over the next three weeks showed trending values eventually leading to critical levels for two measurements. Her white count was low, so we took precautions by avoiding crowds. Even more critical was her platelet level. Three years ago the platelet count reached levels where doctors were concerned about hemorrhaging, necessitating blood and platelet transfusions. We discussed the issue with her oncologist who agreed to forego her next chemotherapy treatment and await further blood test results to prevent any further degradation of the platelet level. Lynne was more lethargic than normal, which affected her speech and ability to get around. Her next set of results show stability and a slight improvement showing that her body was rebuilding after the latest round of chemotherapy.

A week later, Lynne experienced seizures in magnitude that we had not witnessed before, so we made a call to 911 for emergency services. The ambulance took Lynne to a local hospital. The initial CT scan showed no abnormalities and blood test results were stable. The hospital admitted Lynne for further testing. Lynne had an MRI scan and we waited for results. There was some question about the quality of the MRI scan due to Lynne's anxiety causing her to move inside the MRI machine and the lack of appropriate medication to calm her nerves.

The doctors increased her steroid medication, which seemed to eliminate further seizures and improved her speech. My hope was that edema or swelling was to blame rather than tumor enhancement as we were running out of options to address tumor growth. During the process of admitting Lynne to the hospital, Lynne experienced a seizure in her left arm. That was a brand new symptom. This could indicate that the tumor was spreading to the right hemisphere of her brain or simply a factor of edema. Only the results of the MRI scan would shed enough light to understand the cause.

The oncologist received the result of the MRI scan and called me at home. That morning, I was trying to get some work done before heading to the hospital. Lynne's sister, Jessica, and Josh were already there with Lynne. The day we always hoped would be tomorrow came that day. Lynne's MRI scan showed extensive tumor enhancement. No conventional treatments remained. The oncologist said that he appreciated the relationship that Lynne and I had displayed through this ordeal and asked if I wanted to share the news with her before he did. I dressed quickly and headed to the hospital. As I drove, I wondered about the various ways that I would tell Lynne this terrible news. During the first week of Lynne's illness, I told her that I would share what I learned directly, without any sugar coating. She told me that she expected nothing else, so I decided the best way would be direct and short. When I arrived, Lynne and the others had been crying. As I looked down, I noticed that a DNR (Do Not Resuscitate) bracelet was already attached to her arm. Lynne and her visitors did not know why the nurse attached the armband but they must have suspected bad news. I sat down on the edge of hospital bed next to Lynne and reached for her hand. I began sharing the news – the tumor had moved into about 75% of her brain and we were at the end of the conventional treatments. We moved toward keeping Lynne comfortable and ensuring that we filled each day with as much peace and joy as possible. Lynne and I had shared many discussions throughout the journey to prepare ourselves for that day. The discussions helped to ease the transition but only slightly. I prayed with Lynne that she would have an inner peace and that the family would find comfort and strength as we moved into the final stage of the disease.

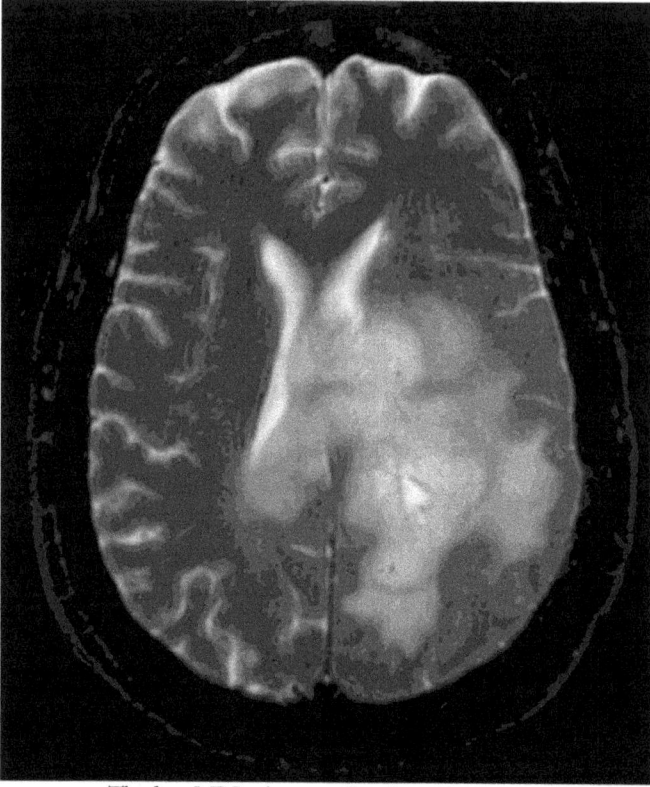

The last MRI taken on October 21, 2010
shows the tumor enhancement and the
crossing of the midline of the brain's
two hemispheres

About one week later on a Friday afternoon, Lynne returned to the emergency room following a precipitous decline in her condition. I was on a business trip to Chicago, so Lynne's sister and Jessica cared for her during my absence. I arrived home from Chicago on an early flight, not yet knowing the news. I received a hearty hug from Lynne and saw her loving gaze that I was very familiar seeing. Not long after, she entered a deep sleep that continued far into the next day. At the recommendation of hospital counselors, I decided to move her to a hospice facility. I now knew that we were in the last days of Lynne's wonderful life. She had touched the lives of many people and for that, I am very grateful.

The day we always hoped would be tomorrow came that day.

Except for brief moments of consciousness, Lynne slept for three days. She was not eating nor drinking. The staff suspended all medications except for three: one to control seizures, one to prevent nausea, and one to manage pain. She was also not receiving anything intravenously. I am thankful that Lynne and I discussed this scenario earlier in her illness. Based on our conversations, I was comforted knowing that the decisions I was making were those she wanted and would make herself. Lynne was resting peacefully. The hospice nurses were very attentive to her needs and provided very good care.

For the next two days, Lynne enjoyed some additional energy. Her friend, Diana, lit up Lynne's eyes at the suggestion of a caramel frappe – one of Lynne's favorite indulgences. At one point, Diana tried to remove the cup from Lynne's hand to warm the hands a bit but Lynne gave her the "stink eye." In other word, "Get your hands off my frappe."

The hospice staff moved Lynne outside for a bit one morning so she could enjoy a little fresh air and the warm sun. She enjoyed the cool air and the sound of the humming birds at a nearby feeder.

She enjoyed visits from family and the many friends she had made over the years. She seemed attuned to sounds, especially to the voices of friends and family. She seemed to recognize many by voice before she did by sight. Despite her condition, she had not lost her caring ways. With each hug that Lynne gave, she added gentle pats on the back with her left arm. One morning, I was outside her room reading some cards sent to her. Some of the cards touched me emotionally and caused me to shed some tears. She heard me and called me into the room where she wrapped her left arm around my back and began her comforting patting. Even in her condition, she mustered the strength to console and provided comfort to others.

A week after her move to hospice, I decided to spend the night at the hospice house as the signs of Lynne's impending passing increased. I was reluctant or simply incapable of resting. The children and I were able to spend some quality time with Lynne that afternoon. I believe she heard our words because she provided some simple acknowledgements. I did notice that she was struggling to focus her vision on those that were speaking to her but I was consoled that she acknowledged their presence in other ways.

On that same day, I made my way to a local funeral home to plan for Lynne's final desires and wishes. Lynne wanted to donate her body for study and research, especially her brain to further the body of knowledge for combating Glioblastoma Multiforme. She also had mentioned in the past that she wanted to contribute to the education of future doctors and possibly to extend the life of someone else. Her caring spirit continued to amaze me. I appreciated her courage. I only hope to build enough courage within myself to make a similar decision.

Saturday, November 6, 2010, at noon, many family and friends were at the hospice facility. Lynne labored for each breath. For two hours, we watched the oxygen saturation levels, which decreased steadily over time. Finally, when the oxygen saturation dropped to 55%, we were sure that she was within just a few minutes of taking her last breath. I placed my head next to hers and held her as I heard Lynne take her final breath. Lynne was a fighter – a fighter to the bitter end.

The family spent an hour with Lynne and comforted one another. The funeral home arrived and waited for the family to complete its goodbyes then loaded her body into a van. They transported Lynne's body to the LifeLegacy Foundation center in Tucson, Arizona.

Three days later, about 400 people gathered for her memorial and celebration of her life. I was grateful to hear stories from friends and family about the many ways that Lynne had touched their lives. Lynne had requested that people donate money to charities rather than providing flowers for the memorial. Many friends and family donated to the National Brain Tumor Society and the Barrow Neurological Institute in her memory.

No language can express the power, and beauty,

and heroism, and majesty of a mother's love.

It shrinks not where man cowers,

and grows stronger where man faints,

and over wastes of worldly fortunes

sends the radiance of its quenchless fidelity like a star.

~Edwin Hubbell Chapin

Chapter 5
From a Son's Eyes

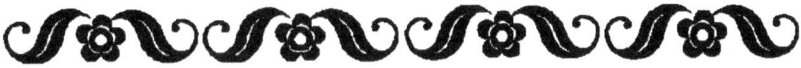

Joshua (Josh), our son, was very close to his mother during his upbringing and they remained close during his adult years. Josh spent many hours and days at the hospital during Lynne's surgeries, recoveries, and rehabilitation stays. Since the preceding chapters discuss the experience from my perspective. I sought out the perspective of Josh and the impact on his life.

For Josh, the diagnosis of his mother was a complete shock. After receiving the news from me, he immediately began asking silent questions within his head, "How could my mom be sick? She was only 46, how could something like this happen to her? The woman who raised me and loved me so much was sick." Thoughts of Lynne consumed Josh's mind – how was she feeling? Josh shared that he wanted only to wrap himself up with her and console her by telling her everything was going to be OK, but oh, if only it was that simple. Josh looked to me for leadership and said that the rest of the family did as well. Josh and the family recognized that I was the one who would research, gather information, and evaluate the options to seek out the best decisions. At the end of the first evening, Josh returned home contemplating ways to face his initial doubt, shock, and denial. He recognized the truth and surety contained within the adage that one minute could change a life forever.

Josh continually reminded himself that he was there to help his mom through this struggle. As a result, he hid his own fears and emotions from her. His daily goal was to make her smile. As Lynne faced many difficult challenges through this illness, Josh continually strove to assure her that everything would be OK. He challenged Lynne to work toward goals and encouraged her as she faced the challenges resulting from brain surgeries. Josh credited his sister and me for their amazing care of his mom. He wished he could have spent more time with her during her illness. He said he would have given anything to spend more time with her. Josh struggled with the balance between existing responsibilities and the new responsibilities that he assumed with Lynne's illness. He regretted the limited time he had to spend with Lynne because of his work. Recognizing this as an unrealistic regret, he still wished to live every waking moment with his mom, for the short time she had left.

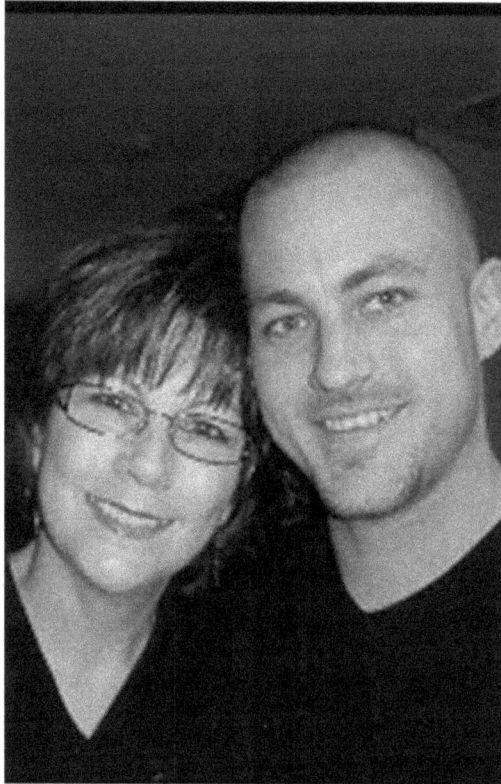

I assured Josh many times that the need for balance is a critical concern for family caregivers. The situation for Jessica and I were just different. To Josh's credit, I recognized his vigil over Lynne during hospital stays and rehabilitation and his weekly visits with his mother and family every Monday and most Sundays despite his long commute. Lynne loved to shop! Josh did too. Lynne enjoyed spending some alone time with Josh as they often spent time getting out of the house. Josh would get her into the car and head to a local store or mall to brighten her day. Many times that was nothing more than a ride in a wheelchair while circling the mall or a favorite store. Josh never arrived empty handed. He normally stopped for a caramel frappe before arriving at the house so he could surprise Lynne with her favorite drink. Josh said he learned a big lesson when facing a dire situation. That lesson: only the little things matter – friends, family, and love.

After his mother passed, Josh spent time researching grief. He learned that people face grief in unique ways and family members react differently to the loss. Josh strove to understand the different emotions each person experienced and the different ways that people recover from grief. He also recognized the different approach that I used versus what he and his sister used, as their approach to grief. Josh shared that we each had different roles within the family and he believes those facts truly pave the road with the means each person uses to deal with grief. As a father, I reminded Josh that he lost someone who is irreplaceable. Although others might fill portions of the void left by the loss of a mother, a person only has one mother.

Josh stated that he struggled about openly discussing the raw emotions that he faced. He shared that he was not one to share and discuss the feelings that swelled within him. His closest group of friends attempted to reach out in kind ways and most of the friends recognized Josh's approach to such an emotional situation. Josh confided mostly with his friend and supervisor Amy. Amy, a friend of 13 years, was the one that would just listen to his cries and screams, and thereby allowed him to discuss his mom's situation openly. Josh received encouraging e-mails and text messages from friends frequently, which he said brightened the present moment. During this trying time, Josh was encouraged just knowing that his friends were thinking about him.

Josh found the most comfort, strength, and encouragement by seeing his mom happy or smiling. Keenly aware of the mortality statistics with glioblastoma, his goal focused on making his mother's last years the most memorable and eventful that he could give. In 2009, Josh planned a surprise 30th anniversary for his mom and me. Josh knew this was a significant milestone for Lynne and me, and wanted to surprise us both. However, the reality of the situation forced him to include me in the planning process. Because too many conversations going on at the same time was hard for Lynne to process, Josh carefully selected a few close friends and family to invite. He arranged to fly in Lynne's parents, from Oregon, to enjoy and celebrate the occasion. I organized a day trip with Lynne, to vacate the house for the necessary preparations. Later that day, Lynne and I arrived back home, Lynne noticed the unusual number of cars parked on the street and remarked, "Someone must be having a party." Under normal circumstances, she would have put two and two together and realized that something was up. I parked the car in the garage and helped her to the kitchen door. When the door opened, Lynne immediately noticed her mom and dad. Surprised, she began to cry. Lynne greeted her mom and dad with hugs, as they hugged the remaining family, and friends filed into the kitchen to complete the surprise. Seeing the surprised look on his mom's face was priceless to Josh. He realized the comfort and joy that Lynne had received by seeing her parents. In much the same way, Josh experienced similar feelings when seeing his own parents.

Josh prepared for grief by assuring his mom that he loved her and wanted to help her be happy. Primary steps, he felt, as those things were the only ones that could help him prepare for her passing. With three years and nine months to prepare, Josh believed he was ready but soon discovered that nothing really prepares somebody to lose a mother. During the last week of her life in hospice, Josh whispered to her that it was OK to go and not worry about the family. He knew his mom had fought a valiant fight and was ready to move on to her heavenly home.

He knew intellectually that his mother could not continue this fight and believed he was mentally prepared for the loss. He soon realized that losing the one person who was genuinely glad to see him and to hear from him every time they saw one another or called on the phone, was a much greater burden than he anticipated. Moments after her passing, Josh went outside asking himself, "What was I thinking?" He was not OK with her leaving us and his major regret was not preparing more fully by seeking the help of a professional grief counselor. Josh held his mom in high-esteem, on the highest of pedestals. He discovered that continuing on, as if everything were fine and normal, was more difficult than he ever imagined.

Josh was 28 years old when he lost his mom. He was just a few years into his adulthood. Josh truly appreciated his mom and genuinely expressed his love for her, sharing that he is a self-professed *momma's boy*. He is not ashamed to say that even in his adult years, he did not quibble about laying his head in his mom's lap. He believes that many people share his major regret of wishing that earlier years had focused on more time with his mom, rather than with friends and other things that teenagers and early adults focus on.

As a father and a *people helper*, I realize that unresolved regrets contribute significantly to the depth of grief a person experiences. Recognizing our human limitations, that our perfect vision of today was mere blindness in the past and learning to forgive ourselves, are key to recovery. In Josh's defense, I recognized his rapid maturity as he faced his newly assumed responsibility throughout the illness. I am thankful that he was at my side throughout the ordeal.

Unresolved regrets contribute significantly to the depth of grief a person experiences

---

When Lynne entered hospice, Josh became very angry. He was angry with himself for taking a business trip the week after learning that no more treatments were available for Lynne and that her life expectancy was about four months. Lynne passed away just two weeks after receiving that news. We learned that there is no guarantee of tomorrow. On the last day of his trip, Josh received a call from his sister explaining Lynne's current condition. After the long flight home, Josh received the phone call from me that he hoped he would never hear – his mom was moving to hospice. At my suggestion, Josh drove home from the airport to rest for the night and met with the family the next morning. Because Lynne slept for most of the week that she was in hospice, Josh believed he missed that last week of her life while he was traveling. In the final eight days of his mom's life, Josh spent 12 to 16 hours each day trying to maximize the time he could spend with her in the final days of his mother's life.

The experience would provide a foundation for Josh to help others experiencing similar situations. Over time, friends and friends of friends contacted Josh to confide in him about life-threatening situations in their own families. They knew he would help by providing a listening and understanding ear. At the time of his mom's illness, he had no friends with a similar experience, so he found that friends were at a loss of words when he tried to share his pain and grief.

I asked Josh to share any advice to friends of someone experiencing a life-threatening situation. He shared that until someone loses a parent, it is difficult to find the right words to offer someone. He suggests that listening and allowing the grieved to talk is helpful. He has found that some people try to contribute suggestions, but until they have experienced the situation, finding the right words to comfort a grieving person is nearly impossible. Therefore, he suggests that people just make themselves available to listen, when the grieving person needs to talk.

Josh believes that one way to keep his mom's spirit and memory alive is to honor her fight. Lynne always wanted to help others. Even after her death, she continued to help others because she planned for the donation of her body and brain for research. To continue her helping ways, Josh joined forces with the National Brain Tumor Society and other causes supporting the fight against brain cancer. Josh became more than just a financial contributor. He joined the planning committee for the Phoenix Brain Tumor Walk. Josh shared that the first experience was extremely fulfilling as he witnessed the host of people completing the Phoenix walk to raise money and awareness for the cause. He was particularly proud to see the large number of family and friends wearing T-shirts emblazoned with a photo of his mom. To walk in her honor was a touching experience. Josh promises to support the cause both financially and physically as long as he is able.

A daughter may outgrow your lap,

but she will never outgrow your heart.

~Author Unknown

Chapter 6
From a Daughter's Eyes

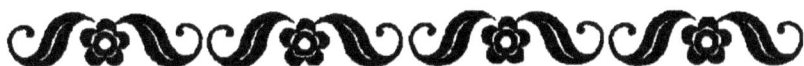

Jessica, our daughter, dedicated most of her time helping to care for Lynne during Lynne's illness. Jessica spent many hours and days at the hospital during Lynne's surgeries, recoveries, and rehabilitation stays. As a result, I sought out Jessica's perspective and the impact of the experience on her life.

Early one morning, Jessica received a call from me saying she needed to get ready and get to the hospital. Jessica asked, "Is there something wrong?" My reply was quick and short, "Just get to the hospital." Jessica pressed me for an explanation, "What is going on?" Jessica's world crumbled immediately at my reply, "They found a brain tumor in your mom," I said, and with that, our phone call ended. Not knowing the full extent of the tumor, her mind raced to the worst-case scenario. As she felt her body go numb, she began to cry. Jessica lay on the bed for a few minutes trying to gather her thoughts. Terrified, she reached for her phone and dialed the number of a family friend. In sharing the news about her mom, she resumed crying, as did her friend. When she regained her composure enough to get ready, she began her drive to the hospital. The six mile, 10-minute drive to the hospital seemed like an eternity. When she arrived at the hospital and located a parking spot, she noticed that her brother had also just arrived. They greeted each other with hugs and tears, both trying to grasp what was going on, and wondering why this was happening.

Jessica and her mom tried to have fun together most of the time, despite the effort it took to care for someone facing a life-threatening disease. Jessica enjoys music and often controlled the selection of music in the car, when she and her mom traveled places together. One favorite memory of Jessica's revolves around a popular song. The song's message focused on the celebration of carefree living, with hands in the air, as though being free from all worldly cares. Each time the song played, Jessica would reach for Lynne's hand; hold it high in the air, waving it back and forth, as she sang the song's chorus. This would make Lynne laugh hysterically every time. When that song plays today, Jessica always remembers her mom's laughter, as well as Lynne's joyous participation in the antics orchestrated by Jessica.

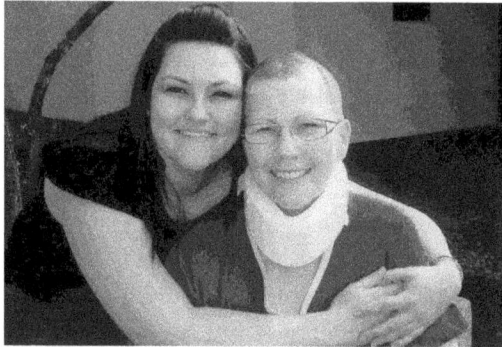

Another memorable thought about the laughs they shared concerns the times that Jessica attempted to serve as the translator for Lynne. When Lynne struggled to piece together a thought, she often pointed toward Jessica. This was her way of requesting that Jessica complete the sentence for her, as though Jessica was a mind reader. When Jessica chuckled and said, "I don't know what you are trying to say, "for some unexplained reason, they would both fall into a hearty round of laughter. On occasion, Lynne did convey her thoughts clearly by her own invented form of sign language. One night as Jessica and Lynne watched television, a cricket sounded off incessantly from the direction of the television. While Jessica ignored the sound as background noise, Lynne's condition caused her to focus on such sounds, Lynne's condition made it difficult to process multiple sounds. Lynne moved her fingers into the shape of a gun, pointed at the location of the cricket, and shouted, "Bang....Bang, Bang." Jessica quickly interpreted the outburst as a command to seek and destroy the cricket. Toward the end of Lynne's life, these types of occurrences occurred more frequently. Reflecting back, Jessica shared that these memories cause her to smile and think about the determination that her mom displayed even during a very difficult time.

Jessica shared the news about her mother's diagnosis with her employer and requested a few days off to be with the family during Lynne's first brain surgery and intensive care unit stay. Her employer told her that he would let her go – not for a few days, but permanently. The termination actually became a blessing in disguise, as it enabled Jessica to help me with the caregiving responsibilities. Lynne needed Jessica more than ever and Jessica wanted to be with her mom during this time. The time Jessica spent with our family helped all of us to grow closer together. Our family supported one another, often without ever speaking a word. We shared a common experience but often reacted in different ways. Jessica recognized that the entire family was terrified about Lynne's condition and about what the future held.

When asked how the situation affected her relationships with friends, Jessica stated, "I found out who my true friends were." Jessica grew closer to some of her friends while she believed others abandoned her. Those who left could not understand what Jessica was going through, and struggled with ways to help her cope. Jessica, like her brother, has learned that just offering to listen is often the best response to a traumatic situation. Many times, no words are necessary - only listening. Friends did reach out to her with e-mails and cards. Some of them came from people she had not talked to in quite a while.

In sharing what provided her with the most comfort, Jessica spoke of her mom's ability to display incredible inner strength, throughout the whole ordeal. Jessica could not recall any instances of Lynne ever saying, "Oh, poor me, I have cancer" nor could she remember Lynne ever even questioning, "Why me?" She simply remembers her mother facing the situation with strength and courage, striving to maintain a positive outlook. Jessica remembers her mother, as the comforter, and when Jessica faced a bad day, she remembers how her mother would wrap her arms around her lovingly, and say, "I love you." Even at the time that Lynne was unable to utter a word, Jessica remembers a certain look from her mom. That was all the "I love you" Jessica ever needed.

To help her prepare for grief, Jessica kept a journal, during most of the time Lynne was ill, recording her thoughts, feelings, and descriptions of Lynne's treatments. Jessica struggled with thoughts about what life would be like, without her mom, and sometimes would call a few friends to talk about the emotions she felt. She would reflect on how different she knew it was going to be, not only for her, but also for her family. Lynne talked with Jessica about the kind of things that Jessica might encounter, once she was gone. Even the times when Lynne could not speak well, she managed to comfort Jessica with these words, "Always be with you." Again, when Lynne could not speak verbally, she always managed to convey somehow the thought, "I love you."

Jessica shared that the work of a full-time caregiver is hard because the stress and emotions take a toll on the body. Jessica shared the regret about showing frustration with her mom at times. Jessica sometimes struggled with the full-time nature of caregiving despite knowing that Lynne found difficulty expressing herself and needed a driver to go anywhere. Despite the intellectual knowledge of these things, Jessica shared about days that Lynne and she would bicker about little things. Most often the bickering ensued when either or both of them were tired and exhausted. Jessica realizes that those little things do not matter over time. Jessica confided that if there were do-overs, she would try harder to let things roll off her shoulders and strive to be more patient. Even in good times, many people hope to be more patient.

Following the terrible news that the treatments moved from fighting the brain tumor to palliative measures, Lynne returned home from the hospital. The next week, Jessica's brother and I had to be away for business. Leslie, Lynne's sister joined Jessica to help with Lynne's care during my business travel. Jessica shared that Lynne slept for most of each day during that entire week. In the middle of that week, Lynne had received a big batch of cookies, which excited her and put a smile on her face. It is amazing how the little things become exciting, when facing the end of one's life. That day, Lynne also managed to muster enough energy to eat lunch with Leslie and Jessica, a highlight for both Leslie and Jessica. Two days later, Lynne became very ill causing Jessica to call for an ambulance.

Once at the hospital, Lynne slept soundly. I was flying home that day from the business trip. Jessica had attempted to call me many times, but had received no answer as I was on the flight. She resorted to leaving me a message to meet them at the hospital as soon as possible. That evening, the doctor told me that Lynne needed to a transfer to a hospice facility. The oncologist believed that Lynne might live another four months, so shock filled each of us, as we now faced this decision. That same evening, Jessica's friend, Sara, arrived from Nevada. She and Jessica had planned this trip several weeks earlier, so they could spend the weekend together with Lynne. Of course, when planning the trip, neither of them realized that they would be spending the weekend at the hospice facility. Jessica, heartbroken at the news of Lynne's transfer to hospice, knew that Lynne was not doing well, but wanted to remain optimistic that her mother would be well enough to return home once again.

After Lynne passed, Jessica said she "felt stuck." Having dedicated over three years of her young life to care for her mother, Jessica struggles to find her place in the world. While trying to adjust to life without her mom, Jessica decided to attend a grief recovery workshop, hosted by a local hospital. Meeting once a week, for 12 weeks, the group followed an approach to the grief process from a book the they read together. The group completed homework assignments each week. Although some homework assignments were difficult, Jessica believes that meeting with the group did help with her grief recovery. Jessica confided, "I honestly don't think the grief ever goes away fully." Jessica shared that she struggles every day with the void left by the death of her mom. Sadness fills Jessica's mind, when she considers all the things that Lynne would miss in her life such as a wedding, grandchildren, the holidays, and family events. Jessica finds some comfort knowing that her mother is always in her heart, and that one day, they will see each other again.

The whole experience has taught Jessica to be able to display empathy for people. Her personal involvement provided her with additional insight into these kinds of heartbreaking situations. She now understands some of the battles that people with cancer face. She is able to share empathy with the caregivers too, because she learned these valuable lessons herself. She discovered that things are much easier to understand, once she had lived through those difficult situations. With the good times and the bad times, Jessica has learned to become a better listener. Sometimes there is no room for words but there is always room for listening.

Jessica and her family have begun to attend the National Brain Tumor walks, in Lynne's honor. Lynne donated her body to medical research and expressed that desire, through her advanced directives. Lynne hoped that the donation would help others through research and provide training, for the next generation of doctors. Jessica contributes her time to these brain tumor walks, which helps to raise money and awareness of this deadly disease, honoring her mom in the process.

I asked Jessica to share any advice to friends with regard to someone experiencing a life-threatening situation. She told me about a response that one person had given to her. That advice consisted of, "Don't feel bad about the situation. Everything is not going to be fun and these are your feelings that you must deal with." Certainly, one could find better advice to share given the situation; however, this helped Jessica to realize that people often struggle with finding the right words to share during a difficult time. Jessica also realizes that the grief process is difficult and life is not always according to plan. Jessica approaches each day striving to remember and think about the happy times.

You don't choose your family.

They are God's gift to you, as you are to them.

~Desmond Tutu

Chapter 7
From the Family's Eyes

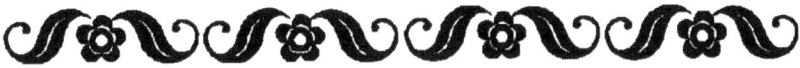

The preceding chapters discuss the experience from my perspective and the perspective of our children. This chapter captures the perspective of other immediate family members. A life-threatening event not only affects the patient but the entire family. Our family members also spent many hours and days at the hospital during Lynne's surgeries, recoveries, and rehabilitation stays. In addition, this life-threatening event also affected friends, although I do not cover those specific topics in detail within this book. I understand that the life Lynne led affected the lives of many other people other than those that I have tried to reference and highlight throughout the book.

Without fail, the initial word used to describe the reaction of all family members upon hearing the news of Lynne's diagnosis was *shock*. Immediately after receiving the news, I called Lynne's parents to inform them about Lynne's diagnosis. For a few moments before the call, I tried to wrap my mind around just how to share such news. I realized that the best approach was to be straightforward. When one of them answered the phone, I asked that they both get together so I would have to share the news only once. I remember hearing sighs of disbelief. Jean, Lynne's mother, later told me the feelings of devastation that she had and remembered the news was hard to believe. Charles, Lynne's father, later shared that he felt overwhelmed by the news. He said, "My beautiful young daughter has a tumor." Charles relied on his religious beliefs and prayed immediately upon hanging up the call that brought the terrible news. He reflected on a biblical passage (2 Corinthians 1:3-4), which reminded him that God is the God of compassion and comfort. Chuck and Jean both made plans to travel from Oregon to Arizona so they could spend some time with Lynne.

Just one year prior to Lynne's diagnosis, my dad received news that he had prostate cancer. A surgery and other treatments placed his cancer in remission but my dad was very familiar with the emotions that surround a cancer diagnosis. Despite the familiarity, my dad said that he felt he was hit with a "ton of bricks" when I shared the news through a phone call. My mother, Sandy, used the word devastated to summarize her feelings about receiving the news. After Lynne's initial surgery and release from the hospital to the rehabilitation facility, my mom flew from Texas to Arizona to spend a few days with the family.

Because Lynne received a neck surgery just one day prior to the diagnosis, Leslie, Lynne's sister, called me from her workplace to see how Lynne was doing. I shared the news about the brain tumor diagnosis. Leslie said after receiving that news, she did not remember the remainder of the call but immediately prepared to leave work and make her way to the hospital to be with her sister. When Lynne's brother, Chuck, received the news, he remembered immediately that he hoped for a misdiagnosis and that life would resume as it had been before.

Some of the immediate family members shared information about the caregiving experience. I asked them to recall any memories that they wished to share. Lynne's father remembered Lynne's positive and uplifting spirit despite the circumstances that she faced. He recalled only a few times when Lynne expressed any sentiments that indicated a depressed attitude. He remembered Lynne's enthusiasm and her happiness to get out of the house – even if it was only for a doctor's appointment. He typically treated her with a trip to McDonald's to fill her cravings and enjoy a caramel frappé. Charles recalled Lynne wondering if she had done anything in her life that brought on the brain tumor. He reassured her that the tumor was not the result of anything she had done but simply the result of living in a world of sickness and disease, a condition resulting from sin entering the world. He shared that Christians do not receive an exemption from that condition and we faced the same disease ridden world as everyone does. Lynne's mother, Jean, also recalled Lynne's upbeat attitude throughout the ordeal. Lynne never seemed to lose her smile. Lynne's attitude made caring for her a pleasure. Witnessing Lynne's determination and fight was encouraging to those who cared for her.

Leslie shared that she had many memories about her care giving experience. She did not share much detail but she did remember the laughs that she and Lynne shared during their visits and when recalling their past together. Leslie fondly recalled sitting with Lynne in silence at times, saying nothing and simply enjoying the time that they had to spend with one another. Like others, she also recalled Lynne's ability to uplift everyone around her. Leslie shared two key words about the experience: forgiveness and love. I am not privy to the details of those conversations between Leslie and Lynne but in a subsequent chapter about grief recovery, I discuss the importance of resolving past issues to ease the grief that results from unresolved issues.

Her brother, Chuck, visited from Oregon two times during Lynne's illness. During Lynne's first surgery, he visited to spend time with her. He recalled a feeling of helplessness, struggling with ways to help Lynne. He tried to fill the void by helping Lynne in any way he could, even with just a simple foot massage. He shared the difficult internal struggle that he had because of the distance between our locations.

My mom and dad also lived far away from our home. They were able to visit on several occasions. Lynne and I celebrated their 50th wedding anniversary by going on a cruise to Alaska with them, along with my brother Terry, and Leslie. That week away from home provided a temporary respite from the regimented schedule surrounding Lynne's treatments, for us all.

I asked the family whether they perceived that relationships changed with other family members and friends. Many of them shared the feeling that relationships changed in some way. Some recalled that friends found it difficult to talk about the situation; as a result, some recalled the distance and separation created with friends and family. They did share that many friends and family sent cards and many received phone calls to encourage them. Some mentioned that knowing friends were thinking about them and praying for them provided a sense of comfort and encouragement. In my discussions with other people, I find this topic a common thread. Personally, I still struggle whether the separation results internally, externally, or from a combination of both sources. However, I do realize that sometimes a separation between relationships does happen. Lynne's brother, Chuck, provide some insight into this topic. He said he focused his efforts on projects around the home as a means to get his mind off the situation. He shared that increasing the distance between relatives reduced the emotional attachment; thereby reducing the potential hurt resulting from any additional losses. However, Chuck did share that he grew much closer to one friend who had experienced a similar situation. The shared, common experience, between two friends, provided an environment to share thoughts and feelings more openly.

My family shared their thoughts about receiving the news of Lynne's move to hospice. Despite holding out hope that Lynne would be spared from death, the news of hospice drove home the grim reality of the disease. We were all keenly aware of the statistics related to survival, but we had heard of others surviving many years so our hope rested in those few exceptions. The family and friends lifted many prayers to God on Lynne's behalf. However, each of us realized that our plans do not always align with the plans that God has for our lives. We also realized that we all face death at some point in our lives, but we seemed ill prepared when that time actually came to face the loss. As Lynne entered the last days of her life, we also recognized that although Lynne had fought with everything inside her to this point, she was entering a phase were the pain and physical debilitations were taking a toll on her will to continue. We began to realize that our own selfishness to keep her in our lives must be overcome. This meant that we had to prepare for her passing so she would be released from the battle against the disease. One painful reality that many of the family faced during the last week of Lynne's life was assuring her that she no longer had to fight and that we were prepared for her for her passing and her return to the arms of her Creator. During private times with Lynne, many family members provided her with that assurance in their own words. I believe that helped Lynne face her final days knowing that we would be OK despite the fact that we would all miss her terribly.

The family's experience with this battle, for one close family member, deepened the compassion for others facing similar circumstances. We are intimately aware of the daily challenges that people face when battling a life-threatening disease. Even before this event in our lives, those in my family demonstrated compassion for other people but I believe this event increased the awareness for each family member.

Following the loss of Lynne, each family member faced the period of grief recovery. As discussed in a subsequent chapter about grief, the experience is unique to each person. As I discussed grief with my family, the realization of this fact became even more apparent. One family member shared that physical work gave him time to sort through the thoughts in his mind to work through the grieving process. He used that time for coming to terms with the loss that he had experienced. Another family member exchanged thoughts with other people using an Internet site geared toward helping people with their grief. Another family member stated that he exchanged a part of the grief with a celebration of Lynne's life and the joy she brought to his life.

As with my son and daughter, I asked the family whether friends had said something they wished they had not said. My mother, Sandy, shared some good insight into this topic. She shared one statement that she tries never to use herself and hopes others will also avoid, "I know just how you feel." She expanded her reasoning for avoiding such a statement by sharing that each relationship is different. Each relationship brings a different level of connectedness. Each person processes the loss in a unique fashion. Therefore, it becomes impossible to know exactly how someone else feels. Although the sentiment of the statement is understood, the statement minimizes the uniqueness of the relationship and the feelings and emotions swirling through the mind of the grieving person.

May the God of hope fill you with all joy and peace as you trust in him, so that you may overflow with hope by the power of the Holy Spirit.
Romans 15:13

I am deeply grateful for my family and their support during Lynne's illness. Each of them helped in some way to ease the burden and to make the last years of Lynne's life more wonderful than I had ever imagined would be possible, under the circumstances. While I did not seek out input from friends who also provided support, I also thank each one of them that helped Lynne and me during this time. I have encouraging memories of my family and friends during this time. Our lives are changed forever by this loss but I believe new paths lie ahead for each one of us. I am thankful for the hope that lies within me – a hope that was demonstrated by many others that served to encourage me during the time. I hope and pray that each person affected by the loss of Lynne finds peace and comfort in every future day that God's sees fit to bless us with, as each day is truly a gift. There are no promises of tomorrow, only our assumptions that we will have another day. With that in mind, I encourage my family, friends, and the readers of this book to enjoy the relationships that you have in your life today.

"I pray also that the eyes of your heart may be enlightened in order that you may know the hope to which he has called you, the riches of his glorious inheritance in the saints,"
Ephesians 1:18

Death leaves a heartache no one can heal,

love leaves a memory no one can steal.

~From a headstone in Ireland

Chapter 8
Grieving

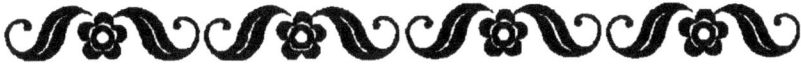

Grief is a universal human experience that will affect every one of us at some point in our life. Although grief is universal, each person prepares for grief, experiences grief, and recovers from grief in unique ways. There are guiding principles that we can apply to our grief but your recovery is unique to your circumstance. You may judge yourself. You might feel as though you recovered from grief too quickly. You might feel as though your grieving is lasting too long. Just keep in mind that your grief is as individual as you are and so is your recovery. It is also natural to believe that others are making judgments about your grief. While that may be the case, your grief is your path, which may look very different compared to the path of someone else.

My grieving process started at the point of Lynne's diagnosis, not her death. The week following her diagnosis, I spent nearly every evening shedding tears and agonizing over the future that lay ahead. Thoughts of unfulfilled dreams and goals circled my mind numerous times throughout each day. As I researched the disease, the certainty of Lynne's eventual death moved to the forefront of my mind. I tried to balance those thoughts with the hope that Lynne's case might be different in some way, but it was a daily internal struggle.

Like any couple, we held onto the hope that our plans for the future would remain intact. We discussed goals throughout our marriage about retirement. We shared about the continued ability to travel. We shared thoughts about the enjoyment of watching grandchildren grow up. We discussed our dreams of a slower paced life hoping to enjoy the simpler things in life. Those kind of things we tend to take for granted in our younger years as we focus on building our lives and careers. In one day, the plans and dreams we made together seemed to shatter like a glass hitting a tile floor. Forever lost with no possibility of ever putting the glass back together.

About six years earlier because of my responsibilities as a deacon at the Sun Valley Church of Christ, I enrolled in a course to help me enhance my skills and abilities as a people helper. As a people helper, people often approached me to share their personal struggles. I desired a better foundation of knowledge to help me guide them through their struggles. A few of the classes within that course of study helped me to prepare for what was ahead in my own life. One class covered forgiveness, letting go of the past and the pain. Another covered marriage and keeping the love alive. Another covered pain and suffering, for learning to help people in a hurting world. Yet another covered managing stress and anxiety. The most important class that would bear on my own future was a class about grief and loss. While my intent was to learn about these topics to assist others, the importance of that learning helped me to understand the emotional turmoil that I was facing and some techniques to help me manage my way through the pain.

Grief is a process that causes psychological pain, creating emotional turmoil with feelings of guilt, depression, anger, sadness, helplessness, rage, loneliness, resentment, and hopelessness. I learned that the emotions that swirled within me were a normal part of the grieving process. Recognizing that early, helped me to be easy on myself as I worked through the grieving process. I believed that I moved to the acceptance phase of the process more quickly than most, in part because of the training I had received.

Another source of strength at that time was my spiritual upbringing and lifestyle. This was also a big part of Lynne's life. With this similar outlook on life, we were able to be in tune with one another. I reflected on one biblical passage frequently, "For I know the plans I have for you," declares the LORD, "plans to prosper you and not to harm you, plans to give you hope and a future" (Jeremiah 29:11, New International Version). Despite this tragedy, I believed that God had a plan. His eternal nature, unrestricted by time, enables Him to see what we refer to as the past, as well as into what we refer to as the future. Time limits me, by allowing me to see only the past and the immediate. Because I cannot see into the future, I reasoned that God could see some future event in Lynne's life that might be much worse than glioblastoma. To me, there could be no worse event but that might simply be due to the limitations placed on me by time and the inability to see into the future.

After Lynne's death, I read a grief recovery book that helped me understand why the depth of grief for one person might be different when compared to the depth experienced by another person. Recovery from grief suggests the ability to recall the good memories you hold fondly while minimizing those feelings of remorse or holding on to the regrets that you are harboring (James & Russell, 2009). I see this as key to understanding the relatively short duration of my personal grieving period.

Lynne and I were very compatible and truly enjoyed our 31 years together as a married couple. We had our fair share of disagreements and disputes along the way. However, we did enjoy a marriage that others recognized in positive ways. The enjoyment of our marriage increased dramatically during Lynne's illness. This may seem very strange to you, so please allow me to explain this phenomenon.

Throughout the early years of our marriage, I appreciated and was grateful for Lynne's concern for others, her willingness to help others, and her support and care for me and our children. Lynne impressed me with her ability to run our home, her industrious nature and attention to details, and a slew of other traits. Yet in the last four years of Lynne's life, I witnessed a courage, vision, and personal strength that I had underestimated in our earlier years together. During those final years, we also discussed topics that most people try to avoid such as death and dying. We discussed what we hoped for one another. She shared her desire that I find another woman to love and care for after she passed. A topic like that may seem like a ridiculous discussion when in health, but it is not whenever someone faces the last stages of life. Lynne shared her appreciation of my care and love for her and her acceptance that I would love and care for another woman in the future. Even before her death, she released me from the anxiety about the considerations about moving on with life, after she passed. In that discussion, she released me from the anxiety or guilt associated with moving forward in life.

Grief Models

While different grief models exist, proposed by many experts, in 1969, Kübler-Ross published the first, widely accepted model of grief. This work provided insight into the emotions that people experience when facing death. Much literature references this model and serves as a basis for discussion, in many articles and papers that followed its release. Later, other researchers extended or revised the model to include other people who experience grief, not only to those facing death. The model suggested a linear progression through the grief. Over time, a growing number of experts rejected the idea that people progress sequentially through the phases. As a result, some experts subsequently provided additional models to help understand grief and the affects that grief has on people.

Like me, you might discover parallels within your grief like those described in the model. Some describe the experience with these grief phases as overlapping at times with some phases extending for prolonged times. I know that grief is not a tidy or straightforward process. Some claim the grief experience feels more like the ball in a pinball machine bouncing from one stage to another with nothing described as sequential. We just need to keep in mind that the way each person experiences grief is unique to the individual. The one huge benefit of these models is that they provide some legitimization for the emotions we experience as individuals as we recover from a significant loss.

Because people reference the Kübler-Ross model most often, I will provide an overview of the following stages:

Shock and Denial

During the shock and denial phase, the shock of the loss is overwhelming. This occurs whether the loss is sudden or anticipated. The griever tends to deny that the loss will occur or has already occurred. This is a normal part of the process for most people. The brain's protection mechanisms help griever's try to cope with the loss.

Anger

Another normal part of grief is the emotion of anger that surfaces because of the loss or the anticipation of the loss. The griever may blame family, friends, or even themselves. The grieved may even blame the person they lost. It is important that the griever express the emotions through sharing with a trusted person to avoid prolonged depression, self-destructive behaviors, health issues, or other negative effects. Depending on the depth of grief, this may lead to a friend, spiritual advisor, counselor, therapist, or physician.

Bargaining

In the bargaining phase, the grieved bargain with themselves, other people, or even with God to avert the loss. The grieved try to seek out options to change the reality of the loss.

Depression

For some, the depression phase is the feeling of sadness or despair, while for others this phase results in clinical depression. It is important to seek out support from a doctor, counselor, therapist, friend, or support group. This phase often leads to other problems, both physical and emotional, if not addressed. For some, this phase is often the longest phase of the grieving process. We pay this price as human beings because we care about others. In any major loss, it is not a sign of weakness to ask for support, in fact, this is an inevitable step, necessary in the grief recovery process. The griever then begins to deal with the often-painful memories and begins to learn to cope with the life changes resulting from the loss.

Acceptance

The acceptance phase results when the pain of the loss begins to lessen. The griever begins to look ahead. The acceptance of the loss causes the griever to move forward, embracing, or at least accepting the changes that the loss created in their lives. The depleted energy resulting from grief begins to increase steadily, as the weight of sadness and despair begin to lift from the griever's shoulders.

Most people move through these phases of grief. The length of time a person spends during each phase depends on the circumstances and is unique to each individual. It is very easy to compare ourselves to other people, and judge that something might be wrong with us, when we do not handle the grief similarly. Just remember, you are unique. Take comfort that your grief recovery is also unique to you. I learned about the grieving process during my studies several years before Lynne's diagnosis and death. That understanding helped me to recognize my emotions and my feelings as well as to accept that they were normal, and to be expected, during a significant loss.

I observed many families over time that lost a loved one. One of the most profound losses a person experiences is that of a spouse because of the relationship depth and the additional potential for economic losses. Based on discussions with those losing a spouse, I believe that losing a spouse affects the relationship within the social circles that the couple shared. I believe there are two contributing factors. First, the surviving spouse draws closer to their own family for support. Second, others within the social circles struggle with the surviving spouse because of the partial loss of identify, that is, the transition from a "couple" to that of a widow or widower. Observations also indicate an increased mortality rate among the surviving spouses, especially in older people because of the major stressor (Gass, 1987, as cited by Harvard Medical School).

In our society, most people recognize the inevitable nature of death but many rarely experience the process because societal norms tend to hide death behind the walls of health care facilities. This tends to deemphasize the process of grieving. This potentially decreases our ability to cope. Sometimes during a terminal illness, a struggle exists between health care providers and families, regarding disclosure of all the facts surrounding the illness. Health care facilities and health care providers maintain various and differing ideologies. This is understandable because some people want the facts and others try to avoid the facts. This simply demonstrates the differences in the ability to cope with illness and the potentially impending death.

Anticipatory Grief

Many patients with terminal illness, and family members or friends who care for them often recognize that death will come eventually. They then begin to anticipate the grief. In the case of Lynne's diagnosis, my research led me to realize the incredible odds against surviving glioblastoma. Despite those odds, I did hold out hope that this case would become an exception, rather than the rule. However, as I reflect back, I realize that I began to anticipate grief while holding on to hope. At some point, I believe Lynne also recognized that the end of her fight was approaching. I believe through her awareness that she helped me prepare for that event. In my case, I believe the anticipatory grief helped me to make the adjustments needed when Lynne passed.

Societal practices try to help people through the grieving process. Funerals provide one such practice. Writing public death notices, writing obituaries, and other traditions contribute to the acceptance of the loss. These help us to face the reality of the loss, which describes a necessary step in the recovery process. Discussing our pain, sharing memories, and sharing experiences help us to face and work through the pain of loss. Recovering from grief includes adjusting to the new environment without a friend, child, parent, spouse, or other loved one. Finally, I hope that we begin to invest anew in our lives while maintaining the memories we have of the one who passed.

With the introduction of the Internet, we discover new ways that people can use online communication and build relationships to facilitate the process of grief. In a later chapter, I discuss my use of technology and the Internet during Lynne's illness. I maintained a blog to facilitate communication with friends and family. The day Lynne died, I posted a message on my blog, and on that same day, over 500 people viewed the message. That post was one-step toward addressing the reality of the loss. As I researched for this chapter, I also located grief forums, where people share their situations with other people, mostly strangers but strangers experiencing the grief caused by a loss of their own. The anonymity, provided by the online forums, supports people in opening up, venting their frustration, anger, and other emotions. It also provides other people an opportunity to show support, encouragement, and provide advice.

Preparation for Grief

Preparation for grief was an important piece of the recovery from my loss. When I say, preparation, you might think that it started during Lynne's illness. I believe that for me, it started much earlier and demonstrated itself in various ways. Because my dad served as a preacher, exposure to death occurred earlier and more often to me than for most young people. Like most, I lived life as if life were going to last forever; however, the exposure to death created an impression on me. The exposure to death helped me to realize that this life is temporary. This mindset helped me to share my appreciation of others before it was too late. Too many times, I heard others speak about their regrets concerning not sharing how much they loved someone or appreciated his or her example until after the death. I feel that is a pity. I decided to ensure that I tried to share my appreciation with those I cared about while they were still living.

Preparation for loss also included setting aside any grudges, anger, bad feelings, and other things that most of us would regret holding onto after the loss of someone close to us. This also includes apologizing to someone for some wrong that we caused. I discovered that stepping up and apologizing when I was wrong was much better than holding onto that wrong eventually causing a regret following the loss of that special person. Avoiding the apology for the wrong might cause regret eventually, following the loss of that special person. This type of preparation averts the regrets we often feel during a loss, whether the loss is sudden, or resulting from a long illness.

Despite the preparation the family and I made, there are areas where I feel we could have improved. Our family digital photo albums date back to 2002 with subsequent albums categorized by year. At Lynne's diagnosis, and through her treatment, the family took about three times the number of photos as in previous years. While photography during an illness may be uncomfortable to some, I am thankful that Lynne was comfortable with the many photos taken of her. One person shared with me that taking photos during the illness, initially seemed strange but later recognized that the family photographs, captured during that time are now the most cherished of all. At the time, I did not foresee the need to collect photographs from others to combine with the family library, but even as I write, I remember some photographs that I can no longer locate. At the time, I underestimated the importance those photographs would have in the future, for helping the family members with remembering important events. I share this as an encouragement to you to collect those pictures and place them in a safe place. You may not realize just how cherished those photos might become.

We captured family videos of the family when the children were young but that decreased over time. I did capture some special moments on video taken while on a cruise with Lynne to Alaska in 2009. I transferred the early family videos from tape format to digital format to make sure that my family could enjoy them long into the future. The family benefits in their recovery by remembering the good times captured in those videos.

Lynne did leave our family some wonderful memories through her scrapbooking. These books not only contain cherished photos but also have Lynne's special touches, as she personally created each page. Several family members and friends have commented that the birthday, anniversary, and 'thinking of you' cards she made for them, still serve as a fond memory of Lynne's caring spirit.

Other areas of preparation included collecting favorite recipes for future use. Lynne was a good cook and an exceptional baker. Her recipe collection was extensive, filling several shelves in our home pantry. We neglected to write down some favorite recipes for the family to share. This is just another area that you might consider focusing on, for storing such information for future use and facilitate the remembering of special times.

You might also collect phone messages and voice recordings. My son has a few phone messages from his mom. One in particular is very special to him. She called Josh to wish him a happy birthday. Unable to take her call at that moment, she left him a voice mail, singing to him. I am unaware of other family members who have such voice recordings but recognize that you might value such a memory in the future. Do consider collecting such items while you have the chance.

For some of these tasks, you might consider asking a family member to help. Your role as a caregiver may be time-consuming, so focusing on tasks like photo or recipe collections might not fit your schedule. When family members or friends volunteer to help, I suggest you consider these types of projects. As a caregiver, you can help other people through their grief by allowing them to participate in some meaningful way. I believe our Creator designed our human nature to serve, so providing opportunities to someone to serve not only helps you but also helps others as well.

Other potential steps exist that help to prepare for the burden of loss. Despite all of the good intentions early in life to prepare a living will, neither Lynne nor I had done so. After her initial brain surgery and recovery, we both prepared a living will and health care power of attorney. Preparing the living will to document Lynne's advanced directives enabled us to discuss Lynne's decisions regarding the end of her life. The health care power of attorney allowed me to represent Lynne when she could not make decisions herself. The discussions we had and documenting them for legal purposes helped me significantly during the final week of her life and the weeks following her death. Knowing that the decisions I made on Lynne's behalf were those that she desired lifted a heavy weight from my heart. The doubts that surfaced in my mind following her death eased slightly, as I knew I was following her desires.

Knowing that the decisions I made on Lynne's behalf were those that she desired lifted a heavy weight from my heart. The doubts that surfaced in my mind following her death eased slightly, as I knew I was following her desires.

In addition, keeping a journal might prove useful during your grief and recovery. Some people incline naturally to keeping journals, while others might struggle with the act of expressing their emotions in writing. For me, writing in the blog and maintaining medical treatment records met only a partial goal of keeping a journal. During the caregiving process of one that is seriously ill, difficult situations arise. Sometimes the experience, and outcomes of the situation will be better and at other times, worse. I believe some people tend to remember these down times because of the protection mechanisms built within the brain. During the grieving process, a journal containing records of the good times we have experienced helps to serve as a reminder for when we experience the sadness that is a natural part of the grief recovery. Recording the emotions you feel during the caregiving process also allows for reflecting back, and I hope, seeing progress compared to how you felt previously. Observing the progress in your own well-being provides an encouragement in its own right.

The many discussions that Lynne and I shared about death and dying during her illness were paramount to my grief recovery. Family members, who openly communicate about death, tend to fare better than families with less open communication (Black, as cited in Carmon, Western, Miller, Pearson, & Fowler, 2010). One reaction to grief is personal growth. This reaction seems most predominant in those that openly communicate about their grief. Other reactions to grief include such things as anger, blame, despair, and panic (Carmon, et al., 2010). The discussions between Lynne and me helped to reduce the uneasiness we held about the dying process. In the final months of her life, I began to sense Lynne's own internal preparation for that day. My selfish nature desired that she live but she showed signs of exhaustion from the three-year battle. As I reflect on those discussions, they are some of my most treasured and valuable memories.

Another preparatory step includes understanding an employer's policies and benefits related to taking time off from work to tend to caregiving and bereavement. Knowing these policies ahead of time potentially reduces the number of concerns and worries, when caring for someone. It also helps when the death occurs. I was fortunate to have a very understanding management chain. However, without speaking to them, I would have increased my anxiety about missing work suddenly or adjusting my work schedule, to accommodate the time I needed to care for Lynne. My two immediate supervisors were very wise. Just days following

Lynne's diagnosis, they scheduled a discussion with me about their intended approach to the situation. This eased my mind significantly, as one thought that crossed my mind during the first week of this ordeal was the potential impact on employment and the ramifications that would ensue.

It is impossible to prepare completely or anticipate all of the emotions and other concerns we face during a loss. I believe that preparing and anticipating the loss causes thinking and actions that help to minimize, if only slightly, the grief of the loss. Reminiscing and expressing emotions with family and friends provide effective coping tools after the death. For me and my hope for you is that the hopelessness turns into hope, and the grief turns into joy, as you learn to push forward and reflect on the positive memories and the legacy of the life that was lost.

Every day may not be good,

but there's something good in every day.

~Author Unknown

Chapter 9
The Brain and Cancer

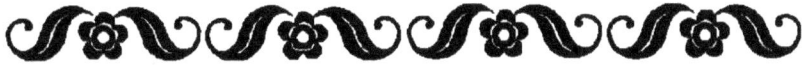

Leaning about brain cancer, in general, and glioblastoma specifically helped me to understand the challenges we would face during Lynne's illness. I spent a number of hours researching the disease for my own benefit but also for the benefit of other people. My first concern was that I have the information to share with Lynne. Second, I wanted the information to share with our family and friends. The knowledge helped to alleviate some of the anxiety associated with the uncertainty about our future. As I learned about the functioning of the brain, this knowledge also helped to explain some of the symptoms and experiences that Lynne faced during her treatments and recovery from brain surgeries. The brain is a complicated organ and central to our being. In this chapter, I will share some of the important information I learned and gathered from doctors, nurses, personal research, and other sources to provide a concise review that I hope benefits you as well.

The Brain

The primary components of the central nervous system are the brain and spinal cord. The human brain, on average, weighs about three pounds. It is a soft mass comprised of nerve cells and supportive tissue. The center of the brain encompasses four ventricles containing cerebrospinal fluid that flows throughout the central nervous system. The brain controls our five senses: hearing, taste, touch, smell, and sight. The brain also regulates emotions, thoughts, speech, coordination, and physical movements.

The brain attaches to the spinal cord, which runs the length of the spine to about the tailbone. Billions of nerve cells, fibers, and supportive tissues support the central nervous system to process messages from the brain to the rest of the body. Some of the messages provide instructions for the involuntary functions of the body such as breathing and blinking the eyes, whereas some process instructions from conscious thought. The skull and the spinal cord protect these fragile components.

We are born with a fixed number of neurons, about 23 billion (Howard, 2006). Some reports suggest that the human brain contains about 100 billion neurons. Regardless, of the actual number, the important fact is the fixed number. In contrast to other cells within our bodies, neurons do not reproduce by splitting to create new cells. Neurons communicate with one another using a dendrite and axon. The dendrite handles incoming messages, while the axon handles outgoing messages. The synapse is a small gap between the axon and dendrite of one neuron and the axon and dendrite of different neuron. Neuron communication occurs over a vast array of connections with other neurons using various chemical compositions. The connections between the neurons define an individual person's characteristics. We learn by creating new neural networks, comprised of synaptic connections and the associated chemical compositions that pass between them. The male brain contains more neurons compared to the female brain but women have more neuropil, the substance containing the dendrites, axons, and synapses that facilitates the communication between neurons. These differences do not contribute to a higher intelligence of one gender over the other; however, some studies do support and explain other interesting differences. For instance, these differences may explain why women appear more adept at multitasking while men appear more adept with spatial reasoning.

The brain contains two hemispheres, the right and left hemispheres. Together, the hemispheres refer to the cerebrum. For most functions, the left hemisphere controls the right side the body, while the right hemisphere controls the left side of the body. Each hemisphere contains four sections referred to as lobes. The names of the fours lobes are the frontal, parietal, temporal, and occipital lobes. Research shows that these lobes are responsible for certain functions or behaviors, for example: emotions, involuntary bodily functions, sight, or hearing. Therefore, the location of a brain tumor or other brain trauma determines the functions potentially affected by the trauma.

The two frontal lobes reside in the front of each hemisphere of the brain. The frontal lobes control functions such as abstract thought, problem solving, judgment, initiative, mood, and inhibition. The two parietal lobes reside in the upper, central portion of the hemispheres. The parietal lobes process physical sensation. The parietal lobes help us to determine the size, weight, texture, and shapes of objects. The parietal lobes also provide spatial processing, that is the awareness of the space around us and the awareness of body parts in relation to one another. The temporal lobes reside in the lower portions of each hemisphere. The temporal lobes process and manage the auditory functions and the translation of words into meaningful information. The temporal lobes also provide the capability for long-term memory. The occipital lobes reside in the back portion of the brain and control vision.

This information that I learned provided the following insight, the brain is an incredible and fascinating organ, with an amazing ability to recover from damage. Even more important than that knowledge, is the brain's ability to retrain itself, following a trauma. Brain surgery, chemotherapy, and radiation damage cells and tissues but the brain demonstrates a remarkable ability for other healthy cells to learn new capabilities that other cells performed earlier. The brain creates new neural networks between neurons to form new communication paths as the brain learns or rehabilitates following surgery. I witnessed this during Lynne's rehabilitation. Following one surgery, the toes on the right foot obeyed the commands given to the right hand. It appeared that communication paths previously responsible for controlling the right hand or foot were learning a new role. It appeared that the newly created communications paths conflicted with each other during the rehabilitation. Eventually her brain worked through the learning process and Lynne recovered most of her function with only limited deficits.

Because I am not a doctor, I will stop with explanations, however, I do want to share that educating myself about the condition helped me to understand some of things that Lynne experienced, and created a more patient and caring advocate. The challenges that Lynne faced required that I be patient and understanding. I also reminded Lynne, that she too, needed to be patient with herself and wait for her body to heal.

Brain Cancer

Having gained a general understanding about the brain, I next researched brain tumors, with a particular focus about glioblastoma. A brain tumor results from damaged DNA that allows cells to divide abnormally. A brain tumor consumes space within the brain interfering with normal brain function and activity. Because the skull, a rigid structure, encases the brain, the tumor increases pressure within the brain by shifting the brain or pushing against the skull. Tumors also invade and damage healthy brain nerves and supporting tissue. The location of the brain tumor influences the symptoms that one might experience, as eluded to earlier. Edema (swelling) within the brain often leads to headaches, seizures, or focal neurological deficits. Focal neurological deficits include movement capabilities, information processing, personality changes, and speech disorders.

Diagnosing

Neurologists perform a neurological examination that spans a variety of tests for evaluation of the functioning of the central nervous system along with physical and mental state. The neurologist evaluates the test results, and may order a brain scan, if any of the results fall outside normal limits.

Imaging technology allows capturing of information about what is going on within the brain. The two most common imaging technologies are the Magnetic Resonance Imaging (MRI) and Computed Tomography (CT). The imaging technology selected depends on several factors. MRI technology uses magnetic waves. This type of technology is avoided for some patients with metal in their body and sometimes for those with tattoos. CT uses ionized radiation and may be limited for patients with a history of x-rays or for children. There are also variations of the MRI technology. The functional MRI maps the brain's activity while performing certain tasks to determine which portions of the brain become active when completing those tasks. This is important when planning surgical procedures, radiation, or other treatments.

When Lynne underwent the functional MRI before her brain surgeries, the technician provided a series of commands during the imaging process. The commands included things like moving the right hand then the left, moving the right leg then the left, and to speak. As Lynne followed the instructions, the MRI collected the images, thus providing insight into the areas of the brain activated by processing the messages resulting from following the commands. The surgeons used the images to plan her surgery and to help balance the risk associated with removing the tumor and minimizing any additional problems. The surgeon also told us that he used the images during surgery to compare the plan with the actual surgical process.

While doctors receive some insight from the imaging technology, the biopsy provides the most accurate method for determining the type and grade of a tumor. A surgeon performs an open biopsy during a craniotomy, which removes of a portion of the skull to gain access to the brain. The surgeon performs a closed biopsy by drilling a small hole into the skull followed by routing a small needle into the desired area to extract a sample of the tissue. A pathologist examines the sample under a microscope to identify the tumor characteristics. The pathologist writes a pathology report describing the findings. The percentage of cells that are dividing provides an indication about the nature of the tumor such as benign or malignant. The higher the rate of proliferation (dividing) also indicates the grade of the tumor.

Causes

One of the first questions that people ask about brain cancer is "What causes brain cancer?" For the weeks following Lynne's diagnosis, family and friends asked this question many times, as they sought answers about the cause of the tumor.

Scientists have conducted and are still conducting many studies into the potential causes of brain tumors. Other than heredity, radiation, and suppression of the immune system, the studies have produced no statistically supported evidence for other causes. Trends do exist but the actual causes are not certain. Research has proven that heredity accounts for only a small number of tumors, therefore, one might assume that other factors are important to consider when trying to understand the potential causes of brain cancer. One focus for research is environmental factors. These environmental factors may include such things like chemicals, diet, cellular telephone, radio waves, and others. As of this writing, little to no proof is available that identifies environmental factors as a specific cause.

Brain Tumor Types

According to the National Brain Tumor Society, there are more than 120 brain tumor types (NTBS, 2011). Scientists often name the type of tumor according to the origin of the cells where a tumor resides. The two types of brain cells are neurons and neuroglia. Neurons process the messages that the brain receives and transmits. Neuroglia supports the neurons by providing nourishment and protection. Pathologists classify tumors using a system that ranges from the least aggressive (benign) to the most aggressive (malignant). Some tumors are associated with a staging classification that indicates the aggressiveness of the tumor. I have learned that despite the classification of the tumor, all brain tumors are serious because they invade such a critical organ, the brain, and prevent normal brain function.

Brain tumors fall into two major categories: primary and secondary. Primary brain tumors originate in the brain, while secondary tumors begin in a different part of the body and metastasize or spread to the brain. Only on rare occasions does a primary brain tumor spread to a different part of the body. Gliomas are tumors that form in the glia cells, the supportive white matter within the brain. Secondary brain tumors are the most common and develop by metastasizing from cancer located elsewhere in the body.

An astrocytoma begins in the glia cells that support the neurons. The astrocytoma is the most common primary central nervous system tumor. A pathologist determines the grade of the tumor ranging from Grade I to Grade IV. Tumors classified as Grades I and II are low-grade gliomas, while tumors classified as Grade III and IV are high-grade gliomas. Low grade means that the tumor grows more slowly as compared to the higher grades, which grow at faster rates. Diagnosing a low-grade tumor often takes longer because the brain adapts to the slow growing tumor. Because of the fast growth associated with high-grade tumors, the symptoms tend to present themselves suddenly and dramatically. Symptoms tend to include headaches, seizures, cognitive deficiencies, behavior changes, weakness in one side of the body, loss of balance, changes in vision, and nausea.

Glioblastoma is a Grade IV glioma. Experts recognize glioblastoma as the most invasive type of glioma, known for its rapid growth, and spread into nearby tissue.

Treatments

The standard treatments, at the time of this writing, include resection, radiation, and chemotherapy. Following the diagnosis, a team of specialists plan and carry out the treatments. The team involves multiple disciplines and specialties like neurosurgeons, neurologists, oncologists, neuro-oncologists, radiologists, and social workers. Rehabilitation following a brain surgery also may require the use of physical, occupational, and speech therapists and depending on the severity of the rehabilitation, the patient may go to an in-patient facility or an outpatient facility.

Some medical facilities use a tumor board to review patient information and collectively reach a decision about the treatment plan. The Barrow Neurological Institute uses such an approach. The approach provided some comfort from knowing that the specialists made decisions using a consensus approach, which by design includes second and third opinions. For our case, this reduced the decision-making time and enabled treatments to begin more quickly. During the seminar that I attended at the Barrow Neurological Institute, two weeks following Lynne's initial brain surgery, I witnessed a mock tumor board with about eight or nine medical specialties represented. The board reviewed a sample case as if they would review any case. I found the process fascinating to watch, as each specialty contributed information from their expertise, then the team finalized their decisions regarding the specific treatment plan. Because each case is unique, the process ensured that each individual received an individual treatment plan based on the needs of that particular patient.

Swelling in the brain (edema) caused by the tumor is one issue that doctors often address before other treatments begin. Because the skull encapsulates the brain, the tumor typically increases the pressure within the brain and the tumor often displaces healthy tissue as it grows. Often, this condition leads to seizures. To minimize the possibility of seizures, doctors prescribe steroids to reduce swelling in the brain. Lynne received various types of steroids throughout her battle to combat swelling and the issues resulting from the swelling. Doctors instruct patients to reduce the use of steroids gradually once the swelling is under control. Tapering off the steroids gradually, prevents withdrawal symptoms associated with steroids particularly if used over an extended time. It is important for the patient to follow the reduced dosing, as per the doctor's instructions.

Surgery is the primary treatment for brain tumors. In some cases, surgery may not be a viable option because of the location of the tumor, and the risks associated with normal brain function. When performing surgery, surgeons carefully balance between removing the tumor and causing additional problems by interfering or interrupting critical brain functions. When possible, surgeons target the entire tumor for removal, though frequently only a portion of the tumor is able to be removed safely. This is referred to as a partial resection or debulking. Even when the surgeon performs a full resection, cancer cells may remain. In either case, radiation and chemotherapy treatments often follow surgery to help kill the remaining cancer.

Radiation therapy uses x-rays or ionizing radiation to interrupt the ability of the cancer cells to divide. Normal cells are better equipped to repair themselves following radiation or chemotherapy than are cancer cells. The hope is that radiation prevents cancer cells from growing again, while healthy cells recover from the radiation and resume their normal function. The radiologist develops a radiation plan that divides the radiation dosage over several applications. Lynne underwent radiation treatments five days per week over the course of about six weeks. The most frequent type of radiation is an external beam that focuses on the tumor location and surrounding area. Whole brain radiation may be used when a patient has multiple tumor sites or for metastatic tumors. Lynne's radiologist provided detailed information about the radiation treatment plan, potential side effects, and answered many questions for us. The technicians provided a tour of the facility and the equipment used, which was helpful in allaying fears about the treatments.

Chemotherapy is another standard treatment for those with brain cancer. Chemotherapy uses chemicals to interfere with the cancer cell's ability to divide and grow. Like radiation, chemotherapy also interferes with the development of healthy cells, but healthy cells recover more readily than do the cancer cells. Surgeons often apply chemotherapy directly to the tumor site during surgery using biodegradable wafers implanted into the tumor site. This treatment is capable of delivering much higher doses of chemotherapy than through other means. The brain contains a built-in protection mechanism referred to as the blood-brain barrier. The built-in protection mechanism helps prevent harmful products from reaching the brain. This same mechanism also prevents some chemotherapy treatments from working on cancer within the brain. The application of the wafers following surgery bypasses the brain's protection system. For other available chemotherapy treatments, oncologists often use a technique that temporarily inhibits the brain's protection mechanism, which allows the chemotherapy drug to enter the brain. Sometimes chemotherapy is unsuitable for some patients because of the individual's health status or sensitivity to the particular drugs. In Lynne's case, her body reacted negatively to several chemotherapy treatments causing the oncologist to halt treatment or find other alternatives.

Chemotherapy often introduces undesired side effects. Most treatments affect the entire body not just the cancer. Chemotherapy interferes with production of healthy cells along with the cancer cells. The way that chemotherapy affects the patients is unique. Additional treatments are available to help the patient overcome some of the negative side effects, such as nausea. Chemotherapy often weakens the body's immune system, as was the case with Lynne. Lynne underwent a blood transfusion and received blood platelets to recover from the damaging effect on her immune system. In that case, the damage to her immune system was severe. Other times, she self-injected a medication that helped to improve the body's production of white cells, those cells designed to fight infections.

This research helped me to consider the options that Lynne faced and provided insight to her when she asked questions. As stated earlier, I attended a seminar conducted by the Barrows Neurological Institute just two weeks after Lynne's diagnosis. The seminar gave me a jump-start concerning the issues we would face during our journey. I do want to remind you that this depth of research fits my personality type. I recognize that other people may not be so inclined to study to the same extent as me; however, I do recommend that you learn enough to help yourself understand the struggles that your loved one will face in their battle.

I ask not for a lighter burden, but for broader shoulders.

~Jewish Proverb

Chapter 10
Caregiver Concerns

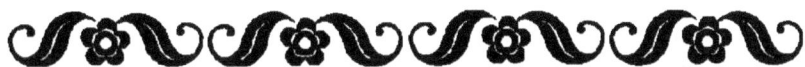

Caregiving is a universal subject. Rosalynn Carter, former First Lady, shared the following from one of her colleagues, "There are only four kinds of people in this world: those who have been caregivers; those who currently are caregivers; those who will be caregivers; and those who will need caregivers."

Some literature suggests that caregivers of patients with high-grade gliomas describe different experiences as compared to caregivers for patients with other types of tumors. Additionally, there is limited information available for caregivers for patients with high-grade gliomas. McConigley, Halkett, Lobb, and Nowak (2010) suggested that the cognitive changes related to high-grade gliomas change the family roles and relationships more rapidly when compared to other types of cancer. Another significant difference is the nearly immediate need for information related to caring for someone diagnosed with a high-grade glioma. The caregiver experiences a substantive increase of responsibility beginning immediately after the diagnosis, surgery, and treatment.

Some caregivers recognized a need to create a new relationship with each other. One that is potentially quite different, when compared to the relationship before the diagnosis. For some, the patient is no longer able to participate as intellectually or physically as before the diagnosis. The location of a brain tumor may also create dramatic emotional changes causing changes in the relationship. The caregivers also find themselves assuming many additional responsibilities that were previously shared or performed by the patient. Caregivers may also find an increased responsibility for decision-making within the relationship. The increased decision-making includes items such as treatments, finances, and routine, practical decisions. Caregivers also face questions about the care to provide and quality of life issues. Even when the patient continues to participate in the decision-making, the caregiver finds an increased need to shoulder the responsibility and help to guide the patient. Caregivers find themselves moving toward an advocate role nearly immediately after diagnosis. This topic is discussed in detail in another chapter.

For Lynne and I, the roles within our relationship began to change immediately following her diagnosis. Following her first surgery, she remained in the hospital for several days then she was transferred to an in-patient rehabilitation facility. Her speech and ability to control the right side of her body were affected significantly after the surgery. She recovered from most of the deficit within a few weeks. In many ways, our personal roles would have been considered traditional. Lynne did the cooking, washing, and cleaning. She also took care of paying the bills each month. I balanced the checkbook and cared for the other financial responsibilities. When she returned home, she could not perform the tasks that she previously performed. The caregiver role included caring for Lynne and also assuming the tasks that she previously attended.

As a result of the shifting roles, the house was no longer as clean as it was before the diagnosis. My family and I ensured the house was clean and presentable, at least most of the time. Because I was able to work from home during Lynne's illness, I multitasked to keep up with the washing. I would start the washer or dryer in between business calls and other work related activities. At first, Lynne was hesitant to relinquish the role of writing the checks to pay the bills each month. She tried to perform the task after returning home from rehabilitation, but the task took about three times as long compared to before the surgery. She finally agreed to transfer the role to me. Lynne preferred handwriting checks each month. To reduce the effort associated with completing the task, I transitioned to using electronic methods that eliminated writing checks. I also setup scheduled bill paying so I could schedule a payment when a bill arrived, providing me the option to perform the task a little at a time, rather than dedicating a larger block of time each month to complete the task. I also discovered that I had a bit of talent in the kitchen. Prior to the diagnosis, my cooking responsibility was limited only to the outside barbeque. However, I found that I enjoyed cooking and preparing meals. When Lynne felt good enough to help, she also enjoyed returning to the kitchen to help prepare meals.

Caregivers also discover the need to learn and gather information immediately after the diagnosis. This can be a struggle because sometimes the caregiver does not even know what questions to ask. With the increased responsibility, the caregivers also need to learn how to take care of themselves. As a caregiver, it is easy to overlook one's own needs. It is important to remember that overlooking your own needs makes you less capable to care for the other person. This might not immediately be the case but over time, your personal strength declines even resulting in health issues of your own.

There is also a need to learn to be a caregiver for a brain tumor patient. This may include managing medications, helping with showers, attending in restrooms, dressing, and other personal care items. Caregivers also face the reality of the patient experiencing seizures. The caregiver must learn how to care for someone experiencing a seizure and learn to discern what warrants emergency care involvement.

In my case, the caregiving experience started immediately following Lynne's diagnosis. The family and I started a round the clock vigil caring for Lynne as she recovered from her first brain surgery, radiation, chemotherapy, and rehabilitation. Lynne's cognitive abilities were not severely affected until later in her illness; however, the physical effects required continual care to ensure her safety. As Lynne was unable to drive, the role of caregiver required coordinating visits to doctors and treatment facilities, and driving her to the appointments. Because the prognosis for patients with high-grade gliomas is unpredictable, the need for the patient and caregiver to make plans about the future and reassess priorities requires immediate attention following the diagnosis. While I strive to avoid minimizing the caregiving experience for other types of cancers, the rapid changes associated with high-grade gliomas normally requires an immediate need for information and caregiving beyond just emotional support to someone diagnosed with cancer.

The National Alliance for Caregiving routinely conducts research to gather statistics related to caregiving in the United States (National Alliance for Caregiving and AARP, 2009). The organization published the most recent report of their findings in November 2009. Nearly 66 million people provided unpaid caregiving services and accounted for about 32% of households. Women assume the caregiving role more frequently than men as female caregivers account for about 66% of the total. About 70% of caregivers care for someone 50 years of age or older. Only about 14% care for someone between the ages of 18 and 49 years. Likewise, about 14% care for children under the age of 18. Caring for someone with cancer affected about 7% of the caregivers. Over 50% of caregivers are between the ages of 18 and 49.

The report determined that the average caregiving experience is between four and five years. About 31% of the caregivers reported that the experience lasted less than one year, 34% reported that the duration lasted between one and four years, and 31% reported the duration lasting five years or more. About four in 10 caregivers reported they believed that they did not have a choice for assuming the responsibility of caregiving.

The report stated that caregivers provide care for about 20 hours per week, when not residing with the care recipient. The hours increase to nearly 40 hours per week when the caregiver resides with the care recipient. About 68% of caregivers stated that other caregivers also contributed to the care but the primary caregivers provide nearly all of the unpaid care. About 17% of the caregivers reported a decline in their own health since the start of the caregiving.

According to the caregiving report, only 15% of caregivers reported a strong financial hardship as a result of caregiving (National Alliance for Caregiving and AARP, 2009). The report concluded that increased financial hardship is associated with caring for children, lower income households, and high burden caregiving situations. The topic of financial considerations are discussed in more depth in another chapter.

Over 70% of caregivers responded that they were employed during the caregiving experience. Of those employed, 66% made adjustments to work schedules by arriving late, leaving early, or taking a part of the workday to attend to caregiving. Only 20% took a leave of absence from their employment. The report stated that employers appear to be increasing their tolerance for flexible work schedules to accommodate employees responsible for caregiving.

I was fortunate in that my work situation allowed me to adjust my work schedule and to work from home. My work schedule moved from a traditional day, where the work hours were performed sequentially, to one where I worked in blocks of time over a longer part of the day.

Learning what you need to know

Only 20% of caregivers reported that they received formal training to perform their caregiving duties. About three-quarters of the caregivers needed more help and information about caregiver topics. The most popular information requests included keeping the care recipient safe (37%), managing stress (34%), and activities with the care recipient (34%), and finding time for themselves (32%)

Things Patients and Caregivers Don't Talk About

Despite the openness of many patients and caregivers to share about the disease and their experience, there are some things that neither patients nor caregivers share with others about the experience. Some of these topics are difficult to discuss, even between the closest of friends. Although these topics are easy to overlook, they are still a common concern for both the patients and their caregivers.

A common side effect of many pain medications is constipation. Constipation is painful and uncomfortable. After about three days, the stool becomes harder and more difficult to pass. Prolonged constipation causes the abdomen to swell, become painful, and can cause vomiting. If this issue arises, discuss this problem with your health care professionals to receive instructions for overcoming or preventing the issue. Lynne experienced one severe bout with constipation following her first surgery. The remedy was painful requiring the nursing staff to intervene physically. I will spare you the details, but rest assured that the experience was not pleasant for anyone involved. Awareness and openness about discussing the issue with doctors and nurses is key for steps to prevent or minimize the issue.

The loss of dignity is also a concern for many patients.

The loss of dignity is also a concern for many patients. As a caregiver, I also recognized the loss of dignity and privacy that Lynne experienced. I tried to ensure that she maintain as much dignity and privacy as possible during her illness. As a caregiver, patient safety was always a primary concern; however, I recognized the need to balance that concern to ensure that Lynne maintained her dignity as a person. Prior to her diagnosis, Lynne was a young person who was fully self-sufficient. I tried to put myself in her place so I could try to understand the emotions that must have swirled within her mind as she was treated and assisted with activities that were otherwise taken care of privately. I encourage caregivers to recognize that caring for the patient's emotional well-being is an important aspect of the process, in addition to caring for the physical needs and well-being. As I researched for this book, I read the writings of another patient. His writings were honest and touching, as he shared his experience. He stated that during the treatments, there was not one bodily entry point that had not been probed, for one reason or another. Often, because of the duration of care following a surgery, the nurses become friends but are still the ones doing the probing and assisting with the otherwise private activities. This causes uneasiness and embarrassment on the patient's behalf. The same is also likely to occur at home when cared for by family or friends.

I encourage caregivers to recognize that caring for the patient's emotional well-being is an important aspect of the process, in addition to caring for the physical needs and well-being

Another concern is the effect of the disease and treatments on one's physical appearance. Surgery causes scars. Radiation and chemotherapy cause hair loss. Radiation can cause burns. Radiation and chemotherapy can also cause other skin irritations. The patient faces often drastic changes in physical appearance following treatments. As a caregiver, it is important to support the patient during these changes. Lynne's head was shaved partially for the first brain surgery. At her request, and rightly so, she wished to keep as much of her hair as possible. Just two days after the surgery, she realized that half a head of hair was probably worse than no hair, so our son, Josh, brought in a set of shears to finish the trimming. Losing her hair was emotional at first but she quickly learned to embrace the new look. Lynne was also concerned and self-conscious about the physical deficiencies she experienced in her right leg following the surgery. While she recovered most of her mobility, she had to wear a brace to help with walking and occasionally she needed to use a wheelchair or walker. Once again, I encourage the caregiver to recognize the emotional turmoil caused by the often rapid changes in appearance and physical condition. Providing positive support is critical to the emotional well-being of the patient.

When facing a serious illness, the desire to just be 'normal' becomes a central theme for the patient.

As individuals, we often strive to be unique and different. For many, the idea of being normal is a little boring in some ways. Humans desire to fit in but at the same time be unique. When facing a serious illness, the desire to just be 'normal' becomes a central theme for the patient. While defining what is 'normal' is difficult or even impossible, the desire to return to a state of normalcy becomes a regular thought. The illness causes changes that the patient cannot control so the uniqueness gained by the illness is troubling. Lynne and I discussed this idea several times during her illness. Together, we tried to define the new normal. We both knew that the probability of returning to the pre-diagnosis normal was very low. However, through our discussions, I believe that Lynne was partially content with the new definition of what was normal for her. This may not be the case for everyone, so the caregiver needs to be aware of this potential concern.

As a new caregiver, I had to learn quickly about the new role. The new role created many concerns that never crossed my mind previously. I assumed new responsibilities. Together, we had to adapt to a new relationship that was foreign to each of us. Our ability to communicate with one another helped with the many new concerns that we faced. While everyone's experience will be unique to their own circumstances, I hope that sharing these concerns helps someone else face the challenges of caring for someone battling brain cancer or other life-threatening illness.

There is no education like adversity.

~Disraeli

Chapter 11
Advocacy

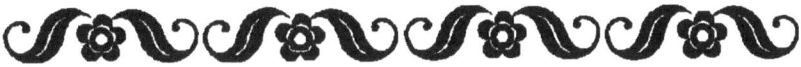

During this caregiving experience, I learned many lessons about the need for an advocate to represent on behalf of the patient. I recognized early after the diagnosis about the importance of this role to ensure the proper care during Lynne's illness. In a sense, I became her case manager to coordinate doctor appointments and all of the follow up care required after surgeries.

During my research, I discovered that many experts recognize the need for the role of advocate for those experiencing an acute illness. The disagreement often arises about the methods for implementing the advocacy role but much less disagreement about the necessity of the role. I witnessed attempts on behalf of the medical community to provide support via an advocate, case management, social worker, along with many other names for the role. Some experts suggest that a close family member not fulfill the role. They suggest that a family member is too close to the situation to provide information objectively. Although I understand that position, I discovered that the attempts of hospital personnel fell short by not providing the continuity of care that Lynne needed. The hospital staff primarily focused on the case for the duration of the hospital stay and faced an inherent conflict of interest (McKinney, 2011). My role as advocate intensified after the hospital stay by coordinating follow up treatments, doctor visits, and facilitating communication between disparate health care providers across multiple heath care facilities. In some cases, I did receive guidance from the hospital personnel to get me headed in the right direction. If you believe you are not receiving the guidance needed, seek out a hospital social worker to help you.

I am compelled to provide some supporting thoughts for a family member fulfilling this role that I learned from my personal experience. The medical personnel fulfilling the role of case manager did not offer to visit our home to determine any needs to assist with Lynne's care after dismissal from the inpatient setting. The hospital discharge instructions rarely considered the factors at home that potentially affected Lynne's recovery. This deficiency required that I bridge the gap as the advocate. As a result, family members and I were in the best position to provide information about the tools that were needed and made available at home. Hospital and rehabilitation staff did question the availability of assisting devices for the home but relied on my feedback as a means of confirming their installation and use at home. To assist Lynne upon her release from the hospital, I installed items like grab bars in the two bathrooms that she used. I purchased a walker with a seat to help her move around the home. I also purchased a bedside toilet that she used, especially when undergoing treatments that often made her nauseated and fatigued. We also removed throw rugs from the floors because Lynne's right foot would drag and catch on the rugs creating a fall hazard. The insurance company or the rehabilitation center provided other items such as a wheelchair, four-legged cane, and gait belt.

Another supporting thought relates to the personal relationship required to understand and fulfill the often complex and wide reaching needs of the patient (Community case managers help navigate health care, 2008). The needs of the patient working through an acute or life-threatening illness extend beyond just medical concerns. I believe that family members who are attuned to the needs of their loved one recognize and fulfill those other needs better than medical personnel that tend to focus only on the medical issues. Because the caregiver spends more time with the patient throughout the illness, I believe the caregiver is better prepared and watchful for other concerns that require attention to ensure the overall well-being of the patient.

The needs of the patient working through an acute or life-threatening illness extend beyond just medical concerns.

During my research for this book, I discovered that the industry of independent advocates or case managers is growing to fill the need of patient representation and provide for continuity of care. If you face a situation of an acute illness within your family, the option may exist to locate a professional medical advocate in your local area. These professionals provide per hour rates and some contract for a flat rate over a specified period. I located some advocates that offer sliding scale rates determined by family income and some even accept cases free of charge (Pro bono) for specific situations.

During the many hours Lynne and I spent at the oncology office for chemotherapy treatments, we had many opportunities to talk with other people about their particular situation. The stories of some saddened me, especially from those facing their cancer alone. While some did not require the same level of advocacy that Lynne required because of the cognitive impacts resulting from brain surgeries, people still need the support of someone that he or she trusts to lean on during the battle. I remember specifically one discussion with a woman undergoing treatments for breast cancer. She shared that her husband had not attended any treatments or doctor appointments with her. The sadness in her eyes as she spoke was heart breaking. I believe that people need to know that they have someone to lean on when facing a traumatic diagnosis and the subsequent treatments.

My research led to the story of a registered nurse diagnosed with lung cancer (Case Management Advisor, 2007). Despite her many years of experience with patient care, she struggled to manage the intricacies of her own care. She shared how the brain seems to freeze, when someone receives a diagnosis of cancer or other acute illness. Even those people with many years of experience in the medical industry discover that navigating the health care system is not an easy task. Discussing treatment options with an advocate eases the decision-making process by providing exploration of options and some clarity about the path forward. The nurse recognized that acute illnesses often require treatment at various facilities and doctors because of the variety of specialties required for treatment. She also shared that the treatment teams often do not communicate and share information with one another effectively (Advocate for cancer patients to help them meet the treatment challenges: case managers help patients navigate through health care system, 2007). Another person described the health care system as fragmented and confusing, especially when facing a serious disease (McKinney, 2011). Even people with health care experience find navigating the health care system daunting and advocating for their own care difficult. Therefore, I recommend someone fill the advocate role to help manage the process and alleviate some of the issues relating to the care of an acute diagnosis.

Another story that I read during my research, discussed the experience of a young woman facing breast cancer (Werner, 2011). As she researched her own situation, she learned that the disease was rare for her age group and tended to be more aggressive in women of her age. She discovered treatment options specific to her situation. However, when she met the doctors suggested by her health plan provider, she discovered the doctors recommended treatments typically provided to older age groups and outdated for women of her age. She eventually located a doctor knowledgeable of the treatments that she had discovered for women within her age group. For all intents, she became her personal advocate. I share the story because sometimes we might feel like victims or passive participants within the health care setting. When in reality, an advocate helps bridge the gap between the health care environment and the patient. While this bright, young lady served the role herself, patients suffering from illnesses that affect cognitive functioning require someone to step up to the task of fulfilling the advocate role.

Lynne's surgical procedures and treatments resulted in stays at four different but local hospitals. I learned that a doctor treating her at one location was unable to see her at another hospital because of the lack of privilege. I learned that hospitals must recognize a doctor and grant privileges to that doctor to see or treat patients. In addition, the hospital provides staff doctors who are often unfamiliar with the history related to an individual patient. In more situations than I care to remember, I needed to step up and share history to prevent the prescription of medications known to affect Lynne negatively. In one case, I rejected the use of one staff doctor for his insensitivity and lack of respect to women. I suspect the issue related to his cultural background, but after warning him twice I refused to allow him to see Lynne in the future because his approach was interfering with her care and recovery. To reference a specific issue, he shared the results of an MRI taken a couple of days after a surgery. He entered her room on a Saturday morning, stated simply and bluntly that the tumor had increased in size then left the room. So for two days, Lynne experienced increased anxiety until she was visited by the neurosurgeon the following Monday. The neurosurgeon assured us both that edema (swelling) resulting from the surgery was actually responsible for the increased size but not because of tumor growth. In my opinion, Lynne was much better off not every seeing that staff doctor again. While situations, such as this one, were rare during our experience, they do happen, so an advocate can help the patient by ensuring respectful and sensitive care from the health care providers.

I also learned that communication networks are limited between hospitals for sharing information about a patient, even by hospitals operating under the same corporate structure. Choosing a particular hospital was an option for some visits but for others the choice was not necessarily ours to make. For instance, there were two neurosurgeons involved with Lynne's care located at two hospitals under different corporations. In addition, during an emergency, the emergency medical services personnel often selected the hospital based on proximity or emergency room backlog. This situation created frustration at times. The situation required that I physically transport records from one location to another, such as MRI and CT scans and associated reports. It became standard practice for me to obtain a compact disc of all MRI scans and the associated reports for our personal records. On multiple occasions, doctors requested that I provide copies to another facility or doctor office. Failing to maintain the records and making them available when needed would have required more scans than necessary leading to additional costs and the unpleasant experience of the MRI scan for the patient.

As an advocate, I also shared treatment history from my own records and notes about treatments received from other medical facilities. I learned that some doctors are very good at requesting the names of other doctors for distributing copies of medical records recorded by the doctor. However, some doctors are not thorough about sharing their notes with other treating physicians. In the story of the nurse, she noted this issue complicated her care, so I know that our story is not unique. Therefore, I recommend that someone fulfill the advocate role to ensure continuity of care and help minimize errors during the treatment process.

I recommend that someone fulfill the advocate role to ensure continuity of care and help minimize errors during the treatment process

As an advocate, I also helped Lynne understand the options presented by doctors for the treatments. Some doctors are better than others are at the task of explaining options. Some assume the patient is cognizant of the medical terminology. Cancer treatments vary depending on cancer type, cancer stage, cancer invasiveness, and different treatment options. I learned that chemotherapy encompasses numerous options and techniques, not one as the singular use of the word "implies." While I was no expert, the brain trauma Lynne experienced caused deficiencies that prevented her from fully understanding the treatment options at times. As Lynne's advocate, I helped her through those decisions by filling the role of advocate.

As Lynne's advocate, I researched resources available in our community and educated myself about treatment options, along with the pros and cons of each treatment. I searched the availability of clinical trials where Lynne met the acceptance criteria. I attended a conference hosted by the Barrow Neurological Institute within weeks of Lynne's diagnosis to educate myself. I also monitored her condition on a continual basis to recognize any changes in her physical or emotional condition that required consultation with a doctor. I helped control the continuity of care required throughout Lynne's illness.

The oncology center that provided Lynne's chemotherapy treatments was often busy with patients. Both patients and the doctor's peers respected the oncologist. In the year of Lynne's diagnosis, the doctor ranked number two of the best oncologists in Arizona as published in a Phoenix magazine. For this survey, the doctor's peers provided the ranking. We believed that we were in good hands with the physician. However, our first few visits to the office were frustrating. Due to the number of patients seen daily, the doctor appeared very rushed during visits. He entered the room, performed an assessment, and then stood while asking if we had any questions. As a new patient, Lynne had numerous questions that often went unanswered at the end of the visit. After a few questions, he moved his hand to the door implying that the discussion was about to end. After two or three visits, I learned to write down the questions ahead of time. On following visits, I would show the doctor a fixed list of questions to ensure him that we had a fixed number of questions. After a couple of visits using that technique, he would enter the room, perform his assessment, and then sit down in a chair while we asked our questions. That simple technique enabled a much better relationship over the remaining years of Lynne's treatment. I suspect the technique demonstrated that we respected his time by preparing for our visits with him. The technique also benefited us by getting the answers to questions and creating a more comfortable relationship with the doctor.

One difficult decision that Lynne and I faced, surfaced early during her treatment and again later in her treatment. The allure of clinical trials and the desperation of one facing a terminal illness potentially look at the promise of the trial for healing. I fully support participating in clinical trials but was selective about the timing. Lynne was young and otherwise healthy at the time of her diagnosis of glioblastoma. Because of these predominant factors; we decided to pursue traditional and approved treatments for Lynne during the early stages of her illness. However, as Lynne's illness progressed we began to consider clinical trials. I provided an overview of clinical trials to Lynne. To gather meaningful statistics and information, clinical trials are tightly controlled and are often performed using statistical groupings to compare the results. Some groups might receive the treatments, while another group receives a standard treatment. This potentially leads to receiving a treatment that is inferior to a standard treatment or missing an effective treatment. This grouping is a necessary part of clinical trials but potentially leads to ineffective treatments, depending on the group assignment. I did not discover any evidence during my research that brain tumor patients receive a placebo, which does occur within some other drug research. After explaining the clinical trials, Lynne understood the risks of participating and recognized the benefit to others down the road. The one clinical trial that we considered, we later discovered that Lynne was not an approved candidate due the number of tumor recurrences she experienced at the time of the trial. It is a courageous attitude for someone to participate in a clinical trial given the understanding that he or she might not benefit directly, nevertheless the patient agrees to continue for the benefit of others and medical research in general. I honor Lynne for her decision and the outlook she maintained about the care of other people.

In addition, as an advocate, I also dedicated much of my time to research about the brain, brain tumors, glioblastoma specifically, potential treatments, and the needs of a brain trauma patient. This armed us with a level of knowledge to help understand the challenges that Lynne would face during her treatments and illness. This knowledge also helped me be more patient with Lynne and be more understanding of the concerns she faced.

Palliative care attempts to improve the quality of life for the patient while suspending further treatments for the disease.

When caring for someone fighting an acute, life-threatening illness, the caregiver potentially faces the decision to transition from treatment to palliative care. Palliative care attempts to improve the quality of life for the patient while suspending further treatments for the disease. This includes preventing or reducing pain and other problems such addressing emotional, physical, and spiritual needs. The caregiver must recognize the need to embrace both medical and non-medical needs. Advocacy seeks to provide the continuity of care for the patient and address the complexity surrounding the level of care needed for the serious illness.

As previously mentioned, a growing industry exists to assist with this need but confusion results by the various names applied to the service, such as case management, care management, care coordinator, care coordination, and managed care. One study suggests that when applied, advocacy increased patient satisfaction. The study also indicated that patients prepared advanced care directives (living will) earlier during the patient's illness (van der Plas, et al., 2012). I assisted Lynne with the creation of her living will shortly after she recovered from her first brain surgery. This provided many benefits to both of us as discussed elsewhere in this book.

The advocate role requires that someone bridge the gap by speaking up for the patient and acting on his or her behalf when needed.

Those facing brain cancers often cannot speak up for themselves. They also may have limited ability to understand the treatment options, pros and cons of treatments, or other information that serves as critical input to their care. The advocate role requires that someone bridge the gap by speaking up for the patient and acting on his or her behalf when needed. This requires that someone objectively evaluates information and, if possible, communicate with the patient using language he or she understands. First, the advocate needs to listen to the desires and wishes of the patient then communicate those desires in positive ways. Second, the advocate needs to understand the various information and advice received by experts or personal research to share them in ways the patient understands. Third, the advocate helps the patient through conflict resolution with other family members or health care providers to ensure the faithful execution of the patient's wishes and desires, especially end-of-life wishes. To fill the advocate role effectively, you must embody good communication skills and a willingness to interface with those in a position of influence and power (Stonehouse, 2012).

While health plans often push for consumers assuming more control for their own care, this is not always feasible, especially for those facing serious and life-threatening illnesses. The need for a family member to assume the role of advocate, or any other name used for the role, is critically necessary to address the myriad of needs for someone facing a life-threatening illness.

*No one can confidently say that he
will still be living tomorrow.*

~Euripides

Death is a distant rumor to the young.

~Andrew A. Rooney

Chapter 12
Legal, Financial, and Insurance Issues

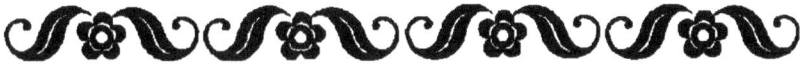

Despite all of our good intentions early in life to prepare a living will, neither Lynne nor I had done so. After her initial brain surgery and recovery, we both prepared a living will and health care power of attorney. The living will documented Lynne's end of life wishes. The health care power of attorney provided me the right to represent her regarding medical issues.

Legal Issues

There are at least two important documents that every adult person should prepare. The first is the living will. The second is the health care power of attorney. Both of these documents came to bear during Lynne's illness. Other documents may also be necessary depending on your particular situation, so consult an attorney to address any outstanding questions or issues related to your situation.

Living Will

If you have not prepared a living will, do your family a favor and get one created. Like many couples, Lynne and I postponed creating legal documents during the years when we were both young and healthy. Luckily for us, we were able to create a living will for each of us soon after Lynne's first surgery. I suspect that as you read this section, you will nod your head in agreement that having the necessary legal documents is important. Upon hearing a newscast or reading an article about the need to create a living will, I did exactly the same thing and promised myself to take the time to create the document. However, it seemed that there was always something else more important to do at the time. After Lynne's diagnosis, I understood the importance of that document. The living will provides written documentation about someone's end of life decisions as related to the medical treatment measures taken to sustain or prolong life during a terminal illness, should one be unable to communicate or become mentally incompetent to make decisions for themselves.

Many people mention these decisions in a fleeting discussion but rarely does someone capture those decisions in writing. Don't think that it can't or won't happen to you because none of us are smart enough or in control enough to know that for sure. There may come a time in life when he or she is simply incapable to convey their individual wishes or desires to allow someone else to act on their behalf. I was fortunate that Lynne recovered to a point where she was able to share her end of life decisions with me. I captured those decisions using a software package that I purchased. At the same time, I also captured my own end of life decisions. After reviewing the documents and agreeing about the contents, we took a short trip to a notary for signatures. The entire process took no more than two or three hours to complete. That small effort and time provided many benefits when Lynne entered hospice just three years later.

One major benefit, for me, was that I became confident regarding the instructions that I passed to the funeral home concerning Lynne's donation to science and the processing of her remains. Those are very difficult decisions to make, and I believe more difficult, if you do not capture the desires of your loved one ahead of time. Another benefit was that I could share Lynne's decisions with other family members if needed. In my case, no family members challenged any decisions that I made but the news covers stories of other families where that does happen. The living will helps to avoid or minimize the effects of any possible contentions among family members at the end of life. I do not tend to second guess decisions that I make. However, many subliminal questions arose during Lynne's final week about the decisions regarding the end of life. The living will helped me to remember that I was following Lynne's desires.

The requirements of the living will vary from state to state so you may need to consult a lawyer to assist you with completing the living will. During my research, I also located several websites that provide the forms customized for each of the states. You may also find the forms located on your state government's website. I located a complete health care planning kit on the Arizona Attorney General website. I used a software package call Quicken Will Maker. The software produced both the living will and health care power of attorney that was suitable for the state of Arizona. I am not endorsing nor recommending that package over any other method for producing the forms but simply sharing the method that I used.

The living will takes affect *only* when one cannot communicate their wishes or becomes mentally incompetent to make decisions for themselves. The living will also names a physician that makes the determination of competence. Once completed, provide copies to your primary care physician and to other doctors caring for the patient. I recommend you keep a list of people receiving copies of the living will so that updates can be provided when necessary. There are also living will registries that allow you to upload the documents and allow health care providers to access the document online.

Health Care Power of Attorney

The health care power of attorney allows you to name an agent who acts on your behalf should you become unable to make health care decisions. The health care power of attorney goes into affect *only* when the person is unable to make decisions and is activated by the attending physician. The healthcare power of attorney enabled me to collect hospital records and discuss Lynne's health status and care with medical personnel.

Selecting an agent or representative to act on your behalf is an important first step. Creating the health care power of attorney requires that you and the agent discuss individual desires related to end of life decisions. Choose an agent that you completely trust, to act on your behalf, when you can not do so yourself. In the case where a decision is not documented, the agent makes decisions based on what he or she believes you desire. That situation is a difficult one for the agent. When the agent is familiar with your values, the difficult decisions become somewhat easier. The agent needs to have the communication skills necessary to seek advice for uncertain situations. As a last resort, the agent makes decisions using good faith in the best interests of the patient. The agent considers topics such as 1) relief from suffering, 2) preservation or restoration of functioning, and 3) the extent and quality of sustained life. These are difficult decisions for anyone, so having a living will in place helps those who make decisions on your behalf.

Completing the living will requires that you discuss your desires with your agent. These discussions are often difficult because they involve a topic that most people in our society try to avoid. The discussions that I had with Lynne were often difficult. In reflection; however, I find those discussions rewarding because they eased the end of life decisions that we faced. When completing the living will, topics such as the use of cardiopulmonary resuscitation, ventilators, feeding tubes, and other medical interventions are documented. One of my most difficult discussions involved guidance about the "Do Not Resuscitate" or DNR. Despite the discussions, despite our values, despite our beliefs, when the time arrived for the implementation of that decision, it was gut-wrenching. I will never forget the look on Lynne's face when she held out her wrist to display the DNR bracelet that was added shortly after receiving the news about the final MRI report.

Power of Attorney

The health care power of attorney focuses on enabling an agent to make health care related decisions. The power of attorney enables an agent to make legal or financial decisions on behalf of the person or the principal. In my case, Lynne and I maintained all financial records in both of our names, so the need for a power of attorney was minimal. As a result, I did not create one. However, your situation might warrant the need to create a power of attorney. The power of attorney is not a standard document, so each one is unique to the person or principal creating one. The power of attorney documents the level of authority that the agent has for conducting business on the principal's behalf. Consult an attorney for details about the power of attorney. Legal forms are also accessible from other resources such as books or the Internet, which may be suitable, depending on the complexity of your particular situation.

Financial Issues

According to the caregiving report, only 15% of caregivers reported a strong financial hardship as a result of caregiving (National Alliance for Caregiving and AARP, 2009). The report concluded that increased financial hardship is associated with caring for children, lower income households, and high burden caregiving situations. The report indicates that those experiencing severe financial hardship are in the minority. We did not experience financial hardship during Lynne's illness. However, during the first week following her diagnosis, I found many unanswered questions swirled within my head about this topic. Some of the uncertainty was far-fetched but the questions surfaced nonetheless.

Research your loved one's Social Security or pension benefits. For some illnesses, government benefits may exist from Social Security, Medicare, or Medicaid. Learn about potential pension benefits and death benefits available from employers. If your loved one is employed, record contact information for those people you need to contact for assistance with disability or pension benefits. Also research the availability of life insurance plans. Ensure that the beneficiaries of the benefits are updated.

Discuss with your loved one about the location of important documents, bank accounts, and any other planning information related to assuming their financial responsibilities. Some information to consider follows:

- Checking and saving accounts; retirement accounts, 401(k) accounts, and other financial accounts

- Location of safe deposit box and key

- Contact information for attorney, tax professional, financial advisor, employer human resources

- Location of important documents: mortgage, life insurance, pension details, will, disability benefits, and employee benefits handbook

Two major expenses, for most families, are automobile loans and mortgages. In our situation, car titles were created in such a manner than either one of us had the legal authority to sell or transfer the vehicles. As mentioned previously, two months before Lynne's death I traded both trucks for a car that Lynne could enter and exit easily. When I traded the vehicles, Lynne was recovering from her final brain surgery so she could not participate in the deal and sign the necessary documents. As a result, the newer car was titled in my name only. Our mortgage and property deed were still in both of our names and required both of us to change the documents in any way. However, the title included wording that conveyed the deed to the other party in case of death. Because I had not reviewed the legal documents for our home in quite some time, I had concerns about the issues related to the home mortgage and deed. That was one item that I did not pursue prior to Lynne's death. When I refinanced the home, more than a year after Lynne's death, I discovered the concern was minimal, because the legal wording in the deed conveyed the home to the surviving party. I encourage you to review the legal issues surrounding the ownership of properties to ensure that no significant concerns surface resulting from a death or incapacity to make legal or financial decisions. Once again, I recommend you consult an attorney if you have any questions related to legal issues resulting from an illness or death.

Another topic related to finances included the filing of federal and state income taxes. Before I begin, I recommend you consult with a tax expert for topics related to your personal tax situation. I am sharing the tax implications only for my personal situation. Your situation might be different depending on your income, medical expenses, and ever-changing tax laws.

During Lynne's illness, I recorded each expenditure related to medical expenses. In my situation, this included only expenses related to medical co-payments for doctor and hospital visits and for prescriptions. While individual co-payments were small in comparison to the portion paid by the insurance company, the expenses added up to a total amount each year that enabled me to deduct medical expenses on my taxes. This deduction also allowed us to deduct mileage driven for medical reasons. Keep good records related to the mileage driven to all medical treatments. In a normal year, the deduction exclusion was significantly below the value that allowed me to deduct medical expenses. While the federal taxes only allowed a partial deduction for medical expenses, my state tax authority allowed a full deduction for all medical expenses. I recommend you keep a close eye on your medical expenses and record keeping, enabling a benefit from a tax deduction if possible.

Insurance Issues

It is important that you understand the applicable insurance plan for physician, hospitalization, rehabilitation, and hospice care. In Lynne's case, my employer provided the health insurance plan. I understood the coverage about routine health care and hospitalization coverage. However, I did not know about coverage for hospice care. If the coverage did not exist, at least I had some time to discuss and plan for other alternatives. Not long after Lynne's diagnosis, I researched the hospice coverage and discovered that the policy did cover hospice care, for up to six months. Though I hoped we would never use that benefit, I could put my mind at ease, knowing the coverage was in place when needed. If the coverage had not been in place, I had time to consider options for that kind of coverage, should we need it.

When dealing with a life-threatening illness, the doctor visits, hospital visits, and surgical procedures results in a large collection of documents ranging from care instructions to insurance explanation of benefits statements. In our case, the paper required storage into three banker's filing boxes, along with some electronic storage. I moved to an electronic filing system during Lynne's illness. Using the electronic filing system, I scanned documents and stored the documents in files on a computer file system. This minimized the physical storage of the documents and enabled easier searching of the documents, when needed, at a later time.

In my situation, the health insurance through my employer provided coverage for much of the related expenses. Even with health insurance, the out-of-pocket expenses for co-payments, medications, and equipment were still significant, but manageable, over the course of the illness. The expenses left uncovered by health insurance exceeded the threshold required to deduct each year when filing federal and state tax returns, which helped reduce the financial impact. For our situation, the health insurance issues were minor compared to other people that I am familiar, who experienced severe financial ramifications from an illness and the resulting health care expenses.

In conclusion, I want to emphasize the need for the living will and health care power of attorney. Life can change in an instant. The documents provide some peace of mind should an unexpected crisis arise. It is also important to understand the other legal documentation that might be required. For the caregiver, record keeping becomes a necessity to ensure benefits, related to life insurance, health insurance, and the filing of federal and state taxes.

Organizing is what you do before you do something, so that when you do it, it is not all mixed up.

~ A. A. Milne

Chapter 13
Organization Helpers

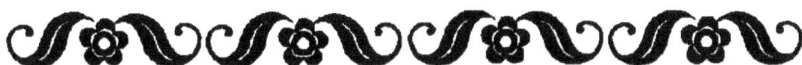

When caring for Lynne, I discovered that organizing information and facts were critical. In this chapter, I will share some techniques that helped me manage all of the information related to caregiving. I work in the information technology industry, so many of the techniques that I used were electronic. The proliferation of mobile technologies today simplifies many of the techniques used for communication, organizing facts, researching, and tracking details.

Communication

The first organization tool helped me with communication. In 2007, about two weeks before the diagnosis, I decided to explore the world of blogging to share ideas unrelated to this circumstance. I set up a blog on BlogSpot to begin my learning process. While I had created the blog, I had not even made my first post to the site before Lynne was diagnosed with brain cancer. Soon after the diagnosis, the blog became an important tool to keep people informed and to reduce my anxiety about the numerous phone calls to and from relatives and friends. As stated previously, we attended a church with about 500 members, so immediately following her diagnosis; I was overwhelmed with calls from family and friends seeking information about Lynne's condition. I often repeated the same information over and over. I decided to rename the blog I had created from its previous name, which I do not even remember anymore, to *The Battle Against GBM*. You can still visit the site at http://darrylpendergrass.blogspot.com/. I set up my mobile device to allow me to post information to the blog wherever I was located at the time. This allowed me the freedom to post information when the opportunity arose and in many cases while the information was fresh in my mind. I directed friends and family to visit the site for the most recent information about Lynne's condition. The blog helped to communicate with more concerned people at one time than would have possible through phone calls or emails alone. I received comments from many friends and family members about the usefulness of the blog to receive timely updates. The blog has received more than 80,000 visits at this time of this writing.

The blog also served to avoid another common problem with human communication. People often use the telephone game story to highlight this communication issue. One person starts the conversation; the next person shares the conversation with yet another person. By the time, the conversation reaches the last person, the original message changed completely because of the multiple misinterpretations and embellishments made along the way. I experienced this firsthand during the early stages of Lynne's illness when I received a call from a panicked relative about Lynne's condition. The relative related that another relative had shared the news of Lynne's impending death. At that point, in the process, besides potential complications arising from surgery, Lynne was not near death. To avoid this issue, I encouraged everyone that was interested to rely on the blog as the *source of truth*.

Another benefit of the blog was the recording of the history of surgeries, radiation, chemotherapy, hospital visits, and the good times that we shared during the experience. The blog also served as a good reference during her care. The blog also helped me remember the timing of events as I began writing this book. As I reviewed the blog, I recognized that I focused on the illness and reporting status much more than I recorded the facts about conversations and other positive memories. In retrospect, I would have been more thorough in recording additional information for the sake of remembering the entire period.

Medication List

A common and frequent question by health care providers was about medications taken by the patient. Secondary in frequency were questions about other health care providers, insurance, pharmacies, past surgeries, and allergies. Doctors often share notes with other doctors to provide a complete picture of the care given to someone. Two organization helpers that I created were a medication list and a health care provider list. During Lynne's care, she often took more than 10 medications with different schedules and used them for different purposes or in combination for a particular issue such as minimizing seizures. The prescribed amount of medication also changed frequently. Trying to memorize such a list would have been difficult and surely led to mistakes when giving Lynne her medications. I simply used a spreadsheet to create the medication list. A sample of the medication list is available for download at the following location.

http://darrylpendergrass.com/books/suddencaregiver/resources.htm

Name	Used For	Instructions	Morning (8:00 am)	Afternoon	Evening (6:00 pm)	Bedtime
Dilantin (100mg and .0mg)	Seizure	Take 100mg morning and evening	100mg		100mg	
Gabapentin 300mg	Seizure	Take 300mg morning and evening	80 mg		30 mg	
Keppra 500mg			x		x	
Levetiracetam	Seizure	Take 1000mg morning and 1000mg evening	XX		XXX	
Lexapro - 20mg	Depression	Take 20mg each morning	x			
Baclofen - 10mg	Spasms	Take 2 tablets each evening			XX	
Clonazepam 0.5 mg	Seizure	Take 1 tablet twice daily	x		x	
Coumadin - 2.5mg		Take 2.5 mg once every other day and 5.0 mg on alternating days	x			
Warfarin	Blood Thinner		XX			
Dexamethasone - 2 mg	Steroid - swelling	Take one tablet each evening			x	
Temazepam 30mg	Sleeping	Take 1 capsule at bedtime				x
Lorazepam 1mg	Anxiety	Take 1 tablet every 8 hours as needed				y
Hydrocodone/APAP 5/500mg	Pain	Take 1 to 2 tablets every 4 hours as needed				

The importance of the medication list was even more important during an emergency. During the illness, we made many trips to the emergency room or had medical services dispatched to the home. Emergency medical responders often look to the refrigerator for this type of information. Possessing an updated medication list reduced the worry during a time of crisis when most people do not think very clearly as the focus is on the immediate needs of the patient.

The list was handy for ensuring that the administration of medications in the proper doses and at the prescribed time. To minimize errors, we purchased a pill holder that held a week's worth of medication for both morning and evening doses. For those medications required more frequently, we simply set alarms on a smartphone. This reduced the possibility of errors given that multiple people might be administering medication. Medication errors account for more than 7,000 deaths annually both at home and medical facilities (Oriental Medicine Journal, 2000). When reading the medicine information sheet that accompanied the Temodar®, I was particularly concerned with reducing errors. Overdosing on that medication by taking more than five days in a row or more than the prescribed amount could be fatal. The sheet also discussed handling of the medication and the risk of opening the capsule. Because the drug inhibits cell growth, the result of absorbing the power, inside the capsule, could be fatal. My concern about errors increased considerably during this time.

Medical Information Worksheet

Another important resource was the medical information worksheet. This worksheet recorded emergency contacts, health care providers, insurance information, pharmacy information, surgical history, medications, and allergy information. During the initial visit with any doctor or to the emergency room, the first barrage of questions included this kind of information. Possessing the worksheet and having it readily available ensured that I did not miss anything critical. In some cases, I simply handed the information to a health care provider so they could copy the information to their own records. I recommend keeping these two records updated at all times. Your stress level will decrease if you have this information updated and handy. A sample file is available to download.

http://darrylpendergrass.com/books/suddencaregiver/resources.htm

I kept these organization helpers in paper form, on my laptop, home computer, smart phone, and eventually a tablet computer. Having the resources readily available in a variety of locations ensured they were there when I needed them. I encourage you to keep similar records to simplify your life and put your mind at ease by having one less thing to worry about.

	A	B	C	D	E	F
1	Date of Birth:		ENTER FULL NAME			
2	Date of Birth:					
3	Social Security Number					
4						
5			Emergency Contacts			
6						
7						
8			Healthcare Providers			
9						
10						
11						
12						
13			Insurance and Pharmacies			

Medication Information

With each medication received, the pharmacy attached a medication information sheet. I kept the latest copy from each prescription in a folder and discarded previous versions. I referred to those sheets often because of the side effects identified with many medications. When Lynne experienced a symptom, I would refer to the medication information sheets to see if the symptom related to a known side effect of one or more of the prescriptions. This allowed me to discuss the findings with doctors. Doctors sought other alternatives for the medication or informed us that the side effect did not represent any major issue.

When I received my tablet computer, I switched to an application called iPharmacyPro. The tool provided similar information that was on the medication information sheet but also provided other useful features. The first benefit is that I had the information available in soft copy form so I did not need to carry around paper copies. Another benefit was the tool provided additional information that was not available on the medication information sheet.

Medical Learning

There were other applications available for the tablet computer, such as WebMD that provided valuable information. For instance, whenever the doctors or nursing staffing that cared for Lynne used unfamiliar medical terminology, I could easily research and read about the information. Visible Body provides two applications. One serves as an atlas of the human body. The Nervous system version provided me the opportunity to learn about the parts of the body, particularly the brain that doctors spoke about during their care. Since I am an analytical person by nature, this fed my need to learn as much as possible about the brain cancer and helped me to understand the situation from a medical perspective. I did not receive compensation by the suppliers for mentioning their products for the tablet and smartphone mentioned in this book. I am just sharing the applications that I found useful.

Journal

In addition to the blog discussed earlier, I also used a journal application called Chapters on the tablet. I used the journal application to record information obtained during Lynne's care from doctor, rehabilitation, and home nurse visits. Much of that information I was unwilling to share publicly on the blog, so having the additional record proved very useful. The application provided a chronological record of that information. On several occasions, I referred to those records to answer questions for doctors, nurses, or therapists.

Mileage Tracking

The mileage tracking worksheet becomes useful at tax time. A patient with brain cancer spends a large portion of time traveling to doctor offices, hospitals, labs, rehabilitation facilities, and other medically directed places. As a result, the miles traveled really added up over the course of a year leading to a possible mileage deduction on the annual tax return. A sample file is available to download. I kept the worksheet on my tablet computer, so I could easily edit the document wherever I happened to be at the time.

http://darrylpendergrass.com/books/suddencaregiver/resources.htm

	A	B	C	D	E
1	Date	Categor	Miles	Description	Notes
2	Mon, Jan 05, 2009	Medical	31	Dr. Z	Surgery Consultation
3	Wed, Jan 07, 2009	Medical	42	Dr. X	Neurologist Checkup
4	Fri, Jan 09, 2009	Medical	25	Dr. Y	Surgery Prework
6	Sat, Jan 10, 2009	Medical	9	Lab	Blood work
7	Wed, Jan 28, 2009	Medical	9	Rehabilition	Speech Therapy
8					
9	Total		135		
10					
11					

You may choose to use the template as a starting point or you could choose another method for tracking medically related mileage. Even if you just keep a notebook in your car to record the miles, you will benefit at tax preparation time by having the information readily available.

Medical Expense Tracking

Another organizational tip is to track your medical expenses when they occur. I use an application called Quicken to manage my finances. The tool easily allows categorizing expenses. At the end of the year, I used the applications capability to generate reports. At tax time, I generated a report with all of the transactions categorized as medical to provide a total amount for the medical deduction on the tax forms. Other applications with features similar to Quicken exist so you have a choice, if you choose to use an electronic expense tracking application.

Another method is to place all medical receipts into an envelope marked with the month and year. This is a little more time-consuming than the previous method but does serve the purpose of providing some organization around the recordkeeping necessary to benefit from a medical deduction to help offset the cost of medical treatments.

Calendar

The calendar is another important organization tool, which is available in paper or electronic form and is useful for remembering appointments. There were periods during the caregiving experience that nine or more appointments were scheduled in a week covering doctor, radiation, chemotherapy, home nurses, and therapists' appointments. Using the calendar effectively freed my mind from holding this information in my brain; thereby, freeing my brain for other more important activities.

Summary

During Lynne's illness, I discovered that organizing the information related to her care provided a means to prevent medical errors and served as a tool to help recall important information when needed. I also discovered that tracking other related information like mileage and medical expenses simplified the tax preparation process each year. The out-of-pocket expenses related to treatments add up over the course of a year and might be easy to overlook at tax time. After getting comfortable with the recordkeeping and organization, I also found that my personal stress levels decreased. That, in and of itself, is a big benefit to the caregiver.

I encourage you to use tools to simplify and free your mind from some of the details of caregiving. Organizing effectively and reducing unnecessary communications allowed me to spend more quality time with Lynne. When she was resting or sleeping, I had time to work, complete school assignments, and other activities that were important to my well-being. During the caregiving experience, it is important to remember that you must attend to your own needs as well.

I try to take one day at a time,

but sometimes several days attack me at once.

~Jennifer Yane

Chapter 14
Caregiver Stress and Burnout

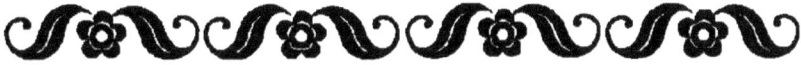

The role of caregiver is a demanding one. Suddenly becoming a caregiver effects many areas of your life and requires reprioritizing and adjustments of other responsibilities. This life-changing and unexpected new role may challenge your health, finances, employment, and relationships. For me, it required learning about a variety of new topics that I never had to consider before this point. I had to reprioritize many things in life to ensure that I had the capacity to fill the role in a manner that would not create regrets later, while still attending to my own needs to minimize the stress associated with the new role. Failing to care for oneself during the process and minimizing stress potentially leads to a mental or physical collapse resulting from sheer exhaustion or burnout. I understand your situation and circumstances will be different but I hope you will gain some insight into the need for establishing priorities to help you with your role as a caregiver.

Work Adjustments

I started to work with Motorola in 1985, so by the time of Lynne's diagnosis I was employed with the company for over 21 years. That situation provided me some flexibility that other people might not be afforded. When I shared the news of Lynne's diagnosis with my management chain, I received support to adjust my work schedule to accommodate my new responsibility as a caregiver. My managers demonstrated true leadership in supporting an employee during a tragic circumstance. I am deeply grateful for the leadership demonstrated by my managers.

My son Joshua received similar treatment from his employer. Joshua received support through his entire management chain, up to and including the chief executive officer (CEO) of the company. Once again, the management demonstrated true leadership in their support of Joshua by allowing him the flexibility to adjust to this new situation.

My daughter Jessica, on the other hand, did not receive similar support. She worked for an orthodontics office. The owner of the office immediately released her when Jessica requested a few days off to be with Lynne. While I understand that he had a business to run, his insensitivity to the circumstances just added additional stress to the already trying circumstance. His lack of leadership and character speaks for itself. I am sure that many people work for similar people, so understand that assuming the responsibility of a caregiver may result in a similar response. Fortunately, Jessica had a savings account that enabled her some time before looking for a new job. However, the United States and global economic downturn that coincided with this time and the resulting effects of losing her mother prolonged her job search several years.

Stress and Burnout

Stress is the body's reaction to a perceived physical or emotional threat (Selye, 1956). Our bodies feel stress regardless of whether the threat is real or perceived. Preparing for the worst-case scenario seems to be a part of our human nature. One major source of stress is fear of the unknown. The uncertainty involved within the unknowns about the future typically generates a large amount of stress for most people. Fear resides in our minds and research supports that most of the fears we conjure up in our heads never becomes reality.

According to Denis Waitley (1983), a study by the University of Michigan revealed that 60% of our fears are totally unwarranted. These fears never come to pass. The next 20% happened in the past. As a result, these fears are out of our control. The next 10% of our fears are those so petty that they make no difference at all to a situation. Of the other 10%, only four to five percent are real and justifiable fears. Half of those fears we can work on and stop worrying about them. Mark Twain said it this way: "I have been through some terrible things in my life, some of which actually happened."

For much of my work career, the companies I have worked for have moved through some significant restructuring, acquisitions, and divestitures. These events generate uncertainty about the future and stress among the employees. As a result, corporations invest heavily in managing the change to reduce employee stress to maintain productivity during the change event. These change management processes typically involve individual or group training and increased communication. A recent training program that I attended included four, one-hour sessions that featured a brain researcher who discussed how the human brain reacts to change and provided some techniques for managing the brain's response to a real or perceived threat. A key learning point from these experiences is that individuals need to recognize stressors, the human response mechanisms, and learn methods for dealing with the stress that is a part of each of our lives.

You increase your risk of stress and burnout when you are the sole caregiver. You also increase your risk if you have complicated family relationships. When you do not receive help from your family, friends, or employer, you also increase the risk of compounding stress. I am grateful that I had several family members and friends who contributed to Lynne's care in various ways and enabled me some time to rest. In the days following Lynne's diagnosis and before her initial brain surgery, several family members converged to help. For the most part, I knew that this help to us would not be permanent, or at least not full-time. I guessed this help would be available for approximately two months. It was difficult and somewhat unnatural but I allowed these family members to contribute as much as possible during that time and tried to maintain my own strength. While other family members would be returning to their homes, I knew that this would be a full-time job for me in the future. When Lynne left the rehabilitation center, following her first brain surgery, she began radiation therapy. The radiation center was approximately 30 miles from our home. Her father volunteered to share the driving, so he and I alternated driving most days. This allowed me to focus on other tasks, while his help was available.

My suspicion about the availability of family and friends tapering off eventually became a reality. I am deeply grateful for the help received during Lynne's illness. I am also thankful that I recognized the need to allow friends and family to contribute to Lynne's care. First, I recognized the need for people to help. People often struggle with just how to help but many people want to help in some way. I admit that discovering ways for people to help was difficult and taxed the mind, at a time when my mind was already disoriented by the diagnosis and assuming the role of the primary caregiver. Creating a list of ways that people can help is useful for the times when someone offers to help in some way. Second, I recognized the need to share the caregiving responsibility as a means to maintain my own physical and mental well-being. I am thankful that I relied on them early in the process, which enabled me to conserve some energy. At the same time, I was able to put in place some changes that helped me to absorb my new duties as a caregiver.

Task Restructuring

One example of restructuring tasks to simplify and reduce time spent on tasks was that of paying bills. Throughout our marriage, Lynne organized and paid the bills. Each month, I balanced the checkbook so I had insight into the family finances but was unfamiliar with the organization she maintained for receiving and paying bills. For a couple of months, I muddled through the process and hoped that some day she would return to health and resume those duties. I considered transitioning from the manual method that she preferred to electronic methods more suited to my style. I hesitated for a few months to see if she could resume the duty at some point. Eventually, she did try to resume the duty, but discovered the responsibility taxed her too much. I eventually converted the management of all bills and payments to electronic methods, which saved me quite a bit of time that was previously spend on that task. I also discovered that the electronic method allowed me to spread out the time needed to complete the task, into smaller chunks of time, instead of a larger block of time just on pay days. When I received a bill, via traditional mail or e-mail, I would schedule the payment and file away the bill. My bank had created electronic bill payment a few years earlier, so the process was fairly efficient by the time that I started using the process. As a

of tasks updated, so that whenever people ask to help, you will have something that they can do to help ease your load as the caregiver.

Balancing short-term stress release techniques with long-term thinking helps you to thrive rather than just survive as a caregiver.

Balancing short-term stress release techniques with long-term thinking helps you to thrive rather than just survive as a caregiver. We often fall victim to focusing only on the urgent rather than the important. Use some of your alone time to reflect on the big picture. As a caregiver, there were times when I fell into the trap of myopic thinking. There were unpleasant and demanding tasks that induced stress. However, striving to maintain a big picture view helped me to keep perspective. Focusing only on the urgent prevents us from seeing the big picture and only serves to increase stress. The big picture view helps you to thrive and not just survive as a caregiver.

Life Balance

In 2005, two years before Lynne's diagnosis, I returned to school to complete my bachelor's degree. This was in addition to working full time. Because of the uncertainty surrounding Lynne's condition and the emotions of the situation, I was unable to focus on school for several weeks. I postponed my remaining classes until I could refocus my efforts. While I struggled to return, I recognized that I was near the end of a major life goal. With the support of Lynne, I did resume about a month after Lynne's diagnosis and completed the bachelor's degree in April 2008.

I recognized almost immediately following the diagnosis that changes needed to occur to create some balance, to ensure that the essentials of life were met. The roles that Lynne previously filled now needed transition to someone else or adjusted in ways, so that our activities were completed, though perhaps not to the same standards as before. I recognized the need to reduce stress and stay healthy, to ensure that I maintained the strength necessary, to care for Lynne.

Tending to your personal needs is not a sign of selfishness. An important part of caregiving is taking care of yourself, to ensure that you will have strength and vitality to care for your loved one. The diagnosis and treatments are a source of stress so additional focus is need to ensure that you manage the stress properly and effectively. The demands of caregiving for a loved one that is seriously ill places additional demands on your life that can take a toll on your physical and mental well-being. Failing to care for yourself makes it harder to care for the one you love.

Tending to your personal needs is not a sign of selfishness.

A challenging part of caregiving is simply reminding yourself to be kind and gentle with yourself in addition to the one you care for. One of the hardest things a caregiver must do is to allow for and compensate for the human element. The human element means that we have limitations as humans. As much as we might admire super heroes, we are not designed to be superhuman. The human element means that we will make mistakes, get angry, get tired, and become frustrated. The human element means that we must remember to be kind and gentle with ourselves. We must listen to the small, quiet voice inside ourselves that reminds us of when we are angry, tired, and frustrated. We must remember to pay attention to our own needs, whether it be for food, drink, rest, or spiritual renewal. To provide consistent love and attention to another, we must first provide it to ourselves because the people who we love and care for depend on it.

My spiritual life contributed heavily to maintaining my mental well-being during this ordeal and to maintaining a life balance. I believe that God has a plan for my life. He had a plan for Lynne's life. I am unable to see the whole plan or even understand it at times. I believe that God loves and cares for me and desires what is best for my life. I am unable to see the entire plan because of my limited perspective. I can only see the past and this very moment. Even then, my personal perspective created by my life experiences often taints my view. As a human with limited perspective, I cannot see into the future. I reasoned that God protected Lynne from something much worse than a brain tumor, despite how difficult that is for me to imagine.

In this life, I also realize that I am not in complete control. Many situations in life are simply outside of my control. I trust that God is in control. That trust allowed me to relinquish the worries and the resulting stress over to Him. That trust helped me to avoid the feelings of helplessness that result during a tragic event. That trust empowered me to focus on the tasks where I did have some control. Peter, in the New Testament, writes, "Cast all your anxiety on him because he cares for you" (1 Peter 5:7, New International Version). Trusting that simple promise, allowed me to reduce stress by realizing that I was not doing this alone.

When performing the duties of a caregiver, stress results as a natural part of the responsibility. Both recognizing the stress and taking actions to alleviate the stress, even if only partially, are needed to reduce the stress to levels that help you maintain your physical and mental well-being. In this chapter, I provided a few examples of ways to help simplify and adjust tasks, to allow the time to absorb the new responsibilities into your life. Remember that taking care of yourself is not a selfish act, but one that renews and reenergizes you to face your new responsibilities day after day.

###

Our own physical body possesses a wisdom
which we who inhabit the body lack.
We give it orders which make no sense.
~Henry Miller

When I stand before God at the end of my life,
I would hope that I would not have a single bit of talent left,
and could say, "I used everything you gave me."
~Erma Bombeck

Bibliography

Advocate for cancer patients to help them meet the treatment challenges: case managers help patients navigate through health care system. (2007). *Case Management Advisor*, 18(4), 37-40.

American Cancer Society. (2009, Dec 17). Irinotecan. Retrieved October 17, 2012 from http://www.cancer.org/treatment/treatmentsandsideeffects/guidetocancerdrugs/irinotecan

Bekar, A., Taskapilioglu, M., Güler, T., Aktas, U., & Tolunay, S. (2012). Effect of Reoperation on Survival of Patients With Glioblastoma. *Journal Of Neurological Sciences*, 29(1), 110-116.

Caretocareprogram. (2012, Aug 29). Caregiver guide. Retrieved October 18, 2012 from http://www.caretocareprogram.com/info/resources/alzheimers-caregivers-guide.jsp?usertrack.filter_applied=true&NovaId=4029462061799202484

Carmon, A. F., Western, K. J., Miller, A. N., Pearson, J. C., & Fowler, M. R. (2010). Grieving Those We've Lost: An Examination of Family Communication Patterns and Grief Reactions. *Communication Research Reports*, 27(3), 253-262. doi:10.1080/08824096.2010.496329

Case Management Advisor. (2007). Advocate for cancer patients to help them meet the treatment challenges. *Case Management Advisor*.

CBTRUS. (2012). Primary brain and central nervous system tumors diagnosed in the United States in 2004-2008. Retrieved from http://www.cbtrus.org/2012-NPCR-SEER/CBTRUS_Report_2004-2008_3-23-2012.pdf

Community case managers help navigate health care. (2008). *Hospice Management Advisor*, 13(4), 45-47.

Falconer, K., Sachsenweger, M., Gibson, K., & Norman, H. (2011). Grieving in the Internet Age. *New Zealand Journal Of Psychology*, 40(3), 79-88.

Genentech. (2012). How avastin is designed to work. Retrieved October 17, 2012 from http://www.avastin.com/patient/gbm/about/index.html

Goldberg, A., & Rickler, K. (2011). The Role of Family Caregivers for People with Chronic Illness. *Medicine & Health* Rhode Island, 94(2), 41-42.

Grieving may trigger heart attack. (2012). *Harvard Health Letter / From Harvard Medical School*, 37(8), 3.

Hamilton, N. (2005). Grief and bereavement: anticipating loss of a spouse. *Nursing & Residential Care*, 7(4), 167-169.

Harvard Medical School. (2011). Beyond the five stages of grief. The bereavement process is seldom linear and varies from one person to the next. *The Harvard Mental Health Letter / From Harvard Medical School*, 28(6), 3.

Howard, P.J. (2006). The owner's manual for the brain. Austin, TX: Bard Press..

James, John W. and Friedman, Russel. (2009). The grief recovery handbook (20th anniversary expanded edition). HarperCollins e-books.

McConigley, R., Halkett, G., Lobb, E., & Nowak, A. (2010). Caring for someone with high-grade glioma: a time of rapid change for caregivers. *Palliative Medicine*, 24(5), 473-479

McDaniel, K. R., & Allen, D. G. (2012). Working and Care-giving: The Impact on Caregiver Stress, Family-Work Conflict, and Burnout. *Journal Of Life Care Planning*, 10(4), 21-32.

McKinney, M. (2011). Empowering the patient: Private advocates help patients navigate complexities of the health system. *Modern Healthcare*, 41(5), 32-34.

Mystakidou, K., Parpa, E., Tsilika, E., Athanasouli, P., Pathiaki, M., Galanos, A., & ... Vlahos, L. (2008). Preparatory grief, psychological distress and hopelessness in advanced cancer patients. *European Journal Of Cancer Care*, 17(2), 145-151.

National Alliance for Caregiving and AARP (2009). Caregiving in the U.S. 2009). Retrieved from http://www.caregiving.org/pdf/research/Caregiving_in_the_US_2009_full_report.pdf

NCBI. (2007, Oct). Interstitial chemotherapy with biodegradable BCNU (Gliadel®) wafers in the treatment of malignant gliomas. Retrieved October 18, 2012 from http://www.ncbi.nlm.nih.gov/pmc/articles/PMC2376068/

NTBS. (2011). Tumor Types. Retrieved from
http://www.braintumor.org/patients-family-friends/about-brain-tumors/tumor-types/

Oriental Medicine Journal. (Spring/Summer 2000). More HMOs covering alternative treatments and complementary care. Vol. 8 Issue 1/2, p11-15, 5p

Pawlik-Kienlen, L. (2009). Caregivers' thrive guide Simple survival strategies. *Alive: Canada's Natural Health & Wellness Magazine*, (318), 78-81.

Pazdur, R.,. M. D. (2011, Nov 18). FDA approval for bevacizumab. Retrieved from
http://www.cancer.gov/cancertopics/druginfo/fda-bevacizumab

Quigley, M., Post, C., & Ehrlich, G. (2007). Some speculation on the origin of glioblastoma. *Neurosurgical Review*, 30(1), 16-20.

Selye, H. (1956). *The stress of life*. New York: McGraw-Hill.

Stonehouse, D. (2012). The support worker's role in advocacy. *British Journal Of Healthcare Assistants*, 6(3), 137-139.

van der Plas, A., Onwuteaka-Philipsen, B., van de Watering, M., Jansen, W., Vissers, K., & Deliens, L. (2012). What is case management in palliative care? An expert panel study. *BMC Health Services Research*, 12163.

Waitley, D. (1983). *Seeds of Greatness*. New York: Pocket Books.

Werner, K. (2011). You're too young for cancer: the unintentional advocate. *National Women's Health Network*.

Zondervan. (1984). New international version Holy Bible. Grand Rapids: Zondervan

About the Author

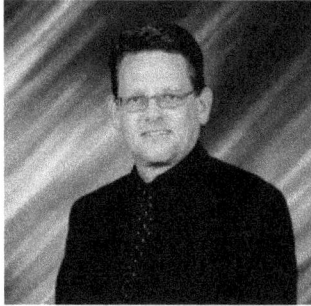

Darryl Pendergrass is a life coach, people helper, and an information technology manager for a large telecommunications networking equipment provider. He earned a Bachelor of Science degree and certificates in general counseling, marriage counseling, and life coaching. In 2007, he became the primary caregiver for his wife who was diagnosed with glioblastoma multiforme – a stage 4 brain cancer. Throughout the nearly four-year ordeal, he received a crash course in caregiving, while advocating on his wife's behalf. He learned many lessons through the experience and shares that knowledge with others in similar situations.

Connect with Darryl

Smashwords author page:
https://www.smashwords.com/profile/view/DarrylPendergrass

Twitter: https://twitter.com/dvpswe

LinkedIn: http://www.linkedin.com/in/darrylpendergrass

Personal Web Page: http://www.darrylpendergrass.com

Facebook Book Page:
http://www.facebook.com/SuddenlyACaregiver

What Others are Saying

"A great legacy that will help someone else bond even closer to their loved one and share together a life-changing trauma. It's not the length of life, it's the quality and hope for the future. You were both winners!" – Tom Finley

"Darryl's faith in God, his faithful love and devotion to his wife of 31 years, and his care for others involved in/with life-threatening health conditions, is readily noticed in the writings of his book. His insight into suffering - hers, his, his family's, and the wisdom he gleaned from it, lovingly blankets the reader with comfort and encouragement." – Joyce Webb

www.ingramcontent.com/pod-product-compliance
Lightning Source LLC
Chambersburg PA
CBHW050128280326
41933CB00010B/1288